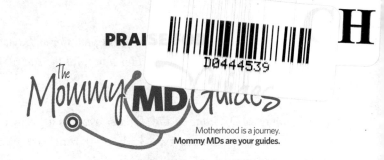

Motherhood is a journey.
Mommy MDs are your guides.

It is fascinating to find the real experiences of physician moms interposed with solid data about healthy pregnancy and delivery. *The Mommy MD Guide to Pregnancy and Birth* is an enjoyable and enlightening book that will "hold hands" with women through their pregnancies.

—*Joanna M. Cain, MD, Chace/Joukowsky Professor and chair, assistant dean of women's health at the Warren Alpert Medical School of Brown University, and obstetrician and gynecologist-in-chief at Women & Infants Hospital, both in Providence, RI*

The Mommy MD Guide to Your Baby's First Year is fun, easy to read, and informative. I love that the advice from physicians is practical and based on experience, in addition to medical expertise.

Since it is a series of vignettes, it's easy to read and pick up in between other activities, which is ideal for busy people like me and new moms.

the medical

Texas

Children's Hospital and an assistant professor at Baylor College of Medicine, both in Houston, and the star of TLC's The Little Couple

❦

The Mommy MD Guide to the Toddler Years is a great testament to the fact that no two kids or parents are exactly alike. I am always looking for new ideas for entertaining, disciplining, teaching, and loving on my kids because what worked with my first child doesn't always work with the other five! I love that this book accepts, appreciates, and addresses the fact that there isn't just one answer to any question or concern parents have with their children. For me, the more suggestions I can get, the better!

—*Casey Jones, a mom of a 9-year-old daughter and 4-year-old quintuplets and costar of* Quints by Surprise, *in Austin, TX*

❦

I found a quiet corner in the living room and flipped open *The Mommy MD Guide to Pregnancy and Birth*, about a topic I last experienced 10 years ago. The more I read, the more I kept thinking to myself, "I wish this book had been *around* 10 years ago." I would have devoured every word if I'd read it 20 years ago, as I plodded through my very first experience with the baffling world of pregnancy. This book really is different from every other pregnancy book I've read.

The Mommy MD Guide to Pregnancy and Birth has

advice from 60 doctors who are moms. Aside from the great medical advice, I was drawn to the anecdotal feeling of this book. As I read, I felt like I was sitting in the living room with these women as they shared their personal stories. I'm a person who loves to hear a good birth story, and I was really drawn to the personal nature of the advice. Instead of feeling like it was coming from a textbook, the advice feels like it's coming from a girlfriend who's just navigated the road herself. But it went beyond "just" a girlfriend's guide, because it was a girlfriend's guide times 60.

I highly recommend *The Mommy MD Guide to Pregnancy and Birth*. I have a feeling many dads wouldn't mind reading it either since it's not long chapters of information, but short snippets of advice, gathered in a very logical way.

I enjoyed the website that's hosted by the authors and look forward to the series this team is working on, covering the other stages of parenting, from newborn sleep issues to elementary school struggles. It's a great idea that was truly done right.

—*Judy Berna, a mom of four and writer for GeekMom.com*

The Mommy MD Guide®

to

Surviving Morning Sickness

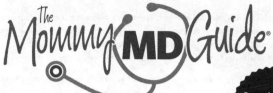

The Mommy MD Guide

Brought to you by the maker of Preggie Pops!

to

Surviving Morning Sickness

More Than 200 Tips That 21 Doctors
Use to Make It Through Morning Sickness
and Related Pregnancy Symptoms

Features GI Pro tips by Stacey Ann Weiland, MD

By Jim Pathman, PhD
and Rallie McAllister, MD, MPH

MOMOSA PUBLISHING

© 2017 by Momosa Publishing LLC

Printed in the United States of America

Book and cover design by Leanne Coppola

Library of Congress information available upon request

ISBN 978-0-9970808-5-8

2 4 6 8 10 9 7 5 3 1 paperback

The Mommy MD Guides®

Motherhood is a journey.
Mommy MDs are your guides.

MOMMYMDGUIDES.COM

To the loves of my life,
yesterday, today, and forever:
my wife, Seana, and daughter, Lanna.
You inspire me, guide me, and make me a better person.
—JP

To my three boys, Chad, Oakley, and Gatlin.
Before you made me so happy, you made me really sick!
—RLM

Contents

Acknowledgments

To say this hasn't been an incredible adventure would be untrue. Being involved with the Mommy MD Guides and Jennifer Bright Reich has been such a wonderful experience in every way. From our initial meetings to the realization of a very valuable resource for newly pregnant moms, is truly a blessing.

There are so many family, friends, and colleagues to thank. I would not even be writing these words if it were not for the genius of my good friend, partner, and colleague nurse Noni Martin. I feel so lucky to have spent the past 20 years working side by side in a Medical Center in Los Angeles. Noni had a dream and a vision to create something that would help new moms feel better, and I was lucky enough to be invited to join her on this mission. She is an outstanding person, and I am forever grateful and thankful to her.

In addition to Noni, three other partners have also been a part of our success over the past 16 years. Joanne, Jeannie and Debbie were there at the beginning and were a constant source of ideas, creativity, and tremendous support.

In addition, I also need to thank my long-time friend, assistant, and right hand, Julie Davine who always has my back and keeps me sane day after day, which has allowed me to be a part of this exciting experience.

Finally, my family has been right beside me as we have lived and loved this journey. From my parents who have always instilled in me the importance of treating people as you would like to be treated, to the joyous support of my amazing wife of 26 years, Seana, and my delightful daughter, Lanna, who would one day love to be a Mommy MD herself.

Thank you all for giving me the honor of being part of this very fulfilling experience. We hope our book has been helpful in understanding some of what you have experienced during your pregnancy and beyond. I wish you joy, excitement, spontaneity, and most importantly an amazing bond with your new baby! There is nothing more magnificent or magical!

—*Jim Pathman, PhD*

The books in the Mommy MD Guides series are proof positive that if we dream big, work hard, and believe in ourselves, we can accomplish anything we feel passionate about. If we're lucky enough to have the help and support of friends and family while we're at it, the process is a whole lot easier, and a lot more fun.

I feel incredibly blessed to have Jennifer Bright Reich as a friend, coauthor, and business partner. Although it's roughly 600 miles from my desk to hers, she's as close to me as a sister. Jennifer and I are both passionate about helping moms carry out one of the most important jobs in the world—raising healthy, happy children. We couldn't do this without the help of our awesome team at the Mommy MD Guides or the incredible physicians who generously share the stories of their lives. I'm grateful to each of them.

I'm grateful to our terrific book team: GI pro Stacey Ann Weiland, MD; copy editor Amy Kovalski; indexer Nanette Bendyna; cover designer Leanne Coppola; interior designer Susan Eugster; writers Jennifer Goldsmith Cerra, Julie Davidson, and Marie Suszynski; proofreader Ashley Kuhn; and printing manager Karen Kircher. Thank you for your efficient, effective, excellent work!

I'm also grateful to my family—Robin, Oakley, Gatlin, Chad, Lindsey, Bella, Cam, and Anna—and very thankful for all the love and laughter we share.

—Rallie McAllister, MD, MPH

Introductions

Congratulations! You're pregnant and about to embark on an awesome adventure. I imagine you are filled with many emotions, from excitement to fear and anxiety. In addition, you may also be dealing with symptoms of morning sickness. With all of these emotions swirling, you may be feeling a little overwhelmed. But hang in there, we're about to offer you some wonderful suggestions and recommendations to help deal with the multitude of feelings that you're experiencing.

For me, when my wife was pregnant, I felt tremendous joy and excitement, but also fear for what possibly lay ahead. We had tried unsuccessfully for three years, so when the news of my wife's pregnancy was finally realized, it was magical. At first, she did not experience morning sickness. (Whew!) But then around the seventh week, she began to have morning sickness—and not just in the morning. It would come and go all day!

My wife coped well with the symptoms, but we searched endlessly for products to help her feel better. It seemed that nothing existed.

As luck would have it, I was fortunate to know and work with my friend and nurse Noni Martin. Noni was an RN and Lamaze teacher. We began to discuss her long-held ideas about a lollipop that could help with morning sickness and could also be used during labor! Well, here we are 16 years later.

Our company, Three Lollies, started with lots and lots of meetings between Noni, Jeannie, JoAnn, and me. It was a wonderful collaboration of healthcare professionals—three nurses and a health psychologist.

As healthcare professionals, our most important mission is to help people feel better. That's why we wanted to be a part of *The Mommy MD Guide to Surviving Morning Sickness*.

My wish for you is that every day of your pregnancy you feel better and better and that as your baby grows and develops, your health and happiness do too! To your healthy, happy pregnancy—and beyond!

—*Jim Pathman, PhD*

When I was pregnant, like so many other moms-to-be, I had that gnawing, disturbing, just-this-side-of-throwing-up feeling of morning sickness. I tried to tell myself it was a blessing—a sign of healthy pregnancy! That didn't make me feel a whole lot better.

Other symptoms that can walk hand in hand with morning sickness down the long and winding road of pregnancy include ptyalism, headache, heartburn, smell sensitivity, and constipation. Will they kill you? No, but they sure will make you uncomfortable!

Just because morning sickness is so common doesn't mean you should suffer through it. There are many ways to ease your discomfort and feel better.

To create this book, we spoke with 21 Mommy MD Guides—doctors who are also mothers. These doctors shared their stories, tips, and tricks about how they made it through morning sickness and its related vexing symptoms.

These smart, funny, fascinating women opened their hearts and lives to us. They shared their challenges and also their celebrations—mainly of feeling good when these stressful symptoms went away.

The more than 200 tips and stories in this book are presented in the Mommy MD Guides' own words, and each tip is clearly attributed to the doctor who *lived* it. Most of these stories contain kernels of advice. This is what doctors who were expecting did to survive morning sickness. Other stories in this book are just that—true stories. The implied advice is: I made it through this pesky problem, and you can too!

Even though this book is filled with advice from a select group—all Mommy MD Guides—you'll find that they hold vastly differing opinions. We've presented many different viewpoints—but not with the intent to confuse or to offer conflicting advice. Instead, these diverse voices are presented so that you can choose what's best for you as you navigate your own pregnancy journey.

As you read this book, keep in mind that every person is different. In fact, every *pregnancy* is different. Things change and improve at different speeds for everyone. Not all progress is the same, and not all progress is linear. You might have some ups and downs. You might experience some plateaus—even some setbacks. Know this: You have plenty of company.

Welcome to the Mommy MD Guides! Best wishes for a terrific pregnancy!

—*Rallie McAllister, MD, MPH*

Chapter 1

Morning Sickness

Considering how common morning sickness is—most pregnant women have at least some nausea, and about a third of them vomit—you'd think we'd know what causes it. Experts think that morning sickness might be caused by lower blood sugar levels or by hormonal changes during early pregnancy. But no one knows for sure.

Despite its name, morning sickness can happen any time of the day or night. Many moms-to-be feel that familiar stomach upset when they wake up, and it often eases as the day goes along.

Morning sickness usually begins during the first month of pregnancy, and it often continues through the 14th or even the 16th week. It usually tapers off completely by the third trimester, but some unfortunate women experience nausea and vomiting throughout their entire pregnancies.

Although morning sickness is making *you* plenty uncomfortable—or even downright miserable— take heart in knowing your baby feels none of this! The only possible concern for your baby is if you have severe vomiting and become dehydrated, or if you lose weight. (See "When to Call the Doctor or Midwife" on page 10.)

It might be comforting to keep in mind that morning sickness isn't a Magic 8 ball. How you feel in one pregnancy doesn't predict how you will fare during future pregnancies.

Some things can make morning sickness worse, such as emotional stress, fatigue, traveling, and eating certain foods. Foods related to morning sickness vary among pregnant women, and they also vary from pregnancy to pregnancy. If you're carrying twins or triplets, nausea in pregnancy is more common, and it can be worse.

One study found that moms-to-be with more morning sickness were more likely to have girls. But don't paint the nursery pink just yet!

JUSTIFICATION FOR A CELEBRATION

One day, you'll wake up, and a few hours later you'll realize you don't feel queasy! Just like that, morning sickness goes away.

> **When you come to the end of your rope, tie a knot and hang on.**
>
> —*Franklin D. Roosevelt*

The first clue that I was pregnant was morning sickness. I noticed that when I brushed my teeth, it made me gag. I bought a two-pack pregnancy test. I took one. It was positive. I took the other one to confirm. It was positive too.

During my second pregnancy, I didn't have any morning sickness. Because of that, I couldn't believe I was pregnant. I probably took 11 pregnancy tests to convince myself that I was indeed pregnant!

When I got pregnant the third time, with my twins, I didn't have to take pregnancy tests. I knew I was pregnant when the morning sickness kicked in.

—*Rebecca Jeanmonod, MD, a mom of 12- and 8-year-old daughters and 11- and 8-year-old sons and a professor of emergency medicine and the associate residency program director for the emergency medicine residency at St. Luke's University Health Network, in Bethlehem, PA*

I think it's helpful to have something in your stomach before you get out of bed in the morning. Some women put crackers on their nightstand.

—*Susan Wilder, MD, a mom of a 22-year-old daughter and twin 17-year-old girls, a primary care physician, and the founder and CEO of LifeScape Premier LLC, in Scottsdale, AZ*

My first pregnancy was a dream! It was absolutely fantastic! I didn't have any morning sickness.

With this pregnancy, I could hardly get out of bed during the first trimester! Morning sickness started around week six. I was so nauseated that I could hardly eat or take my prenatal vitamins. It was difficult even to drink water. I was subsisting on orange Gatorade—not yellow or purple. You don't want to throw up purple Gatorade! Finally around week 14, I turned the corner. Now I feel markedly, 1,000 times better. I can eat and drink again.

—Michelle Davis-Dash, MD, a mom of a five-year-old son, who's expecting another baby, and a pediatrician in Baltimore, MD

When I had morning sickness, traditional food remedies, such as ginger and lemon didn't help. Unfortunately vanilla ice cream sometimes did. I gained 40 pounds!

—Amy Baxter, MD, a mom of 18- and 16-year-old sons and a 14-year-old daughter; the CEO of buzzy4shots. com; and the director of emergency research, Scottish Rite, of Children's Healthcare of Atlanta

Back in my day, we all ate saltine crackers to combat morning sickness. That was very much in vogue. The idea was if you snacked on saltines, your stomach would never be completely empty, and that was supposed to quell the nausea.

—Eva Ritvo, MD, a mom of 25- and 21-year-old daughters, a psychiatrist, and the founder of bekindr.com, a movement to bring more kindness to the world, using neuroscience as the foundation, in Miami Beach, FL

When I had morning sickness, I always had to be munching on something carby. This was especially important when I was driving because that was when my nausea was the worst.

I tried everything—from gingersnaps to ginger candies to chewing gum. Crackers were often the most helpful food.

—*Nilong Parikh Vyas, MD, MPH, a mom of seven- and five-year-old sons and the founder and owner of Sleepless in NOLA sleep consulting, in New Orleans, LA*

When you have morning sickness, you start to figure out which foods you can eat and which you can't. I tolerated salty carbs the best—things like Pringles potato chips and tater tots. I don't usually eat that stuff, but there's something soothing about carbohydrates. Anyone who's ever been on a low-carb diet knows that when you finally eat pasta again, it is deeply satisfying.

As an emergency physician, I work a lot of odd hours. I know that my female colleagues and I often crave salty carbs at night after a shift.

After you've been up all night, you're so tired that you can't tell if you're hungry, exhausted, cold, hot, or what. You just know you don't feel well. In times like that, a lot of women soothe themselves by eating carbs.

—*Rebecca Jeanmonod, MD*

I experienced some morning sickness with both of my pregnancies. The nausea started after a few weeks, and it lasted for several months. Morning sickness is variable. It differs a lot from one woman to another and even from one pregnancy to another in the same woman. Mine was pretty mild, but it lasted all day.

The two things that seemed to help were distraction and eating. A pregnant stomach does not like to be hungry! I worked professionally throughout my pregnancies and found that demands on my attention pushed my symptoms into the background.

—*Elizabeth Berger, MD, MPhil, a mom of two grown children, a grandmother of two, a clinical associate professor of psychiatry at George Washington University, and the author of Raising Kids with Character, in New York City*

Like most pregnant moms, my morning sickness occurred during the first trimester and in the mornings. While my symptoms were mild, I did avoid breakfast for several hours, waiting for the wave of nausea to pass. By mid-morning, my symptoms did improve, and I was able to "advance diet as tolerated," as they say in medicine.

I didn't throw up. But I did some dry heaving, which oddly did improve my nausea.

There is a protective evolutionary theory for morning sickness. During the first trimester, the process of embryogenesis is most sensitive to teratogens. And it's been proposed that maternal morning sickness, sensitivity to smells/tastes helps ensure that mom avoids consuming harmful foods. This theory would also explain why the majority of morning sickness improves by the end of the first trimester. By then, the majority of organogenesis and the baby is more resilient to potential teratogens.

—*Edna Ma, MD, a mom of a 4-year-old son and an 18-month-old daughter, an anesthesiologist, and the founder of BareEASE pre-waxing numbing kit, in Los Angeles, CA*

Dr. Jim's Tip
ARE YOU SERIOUS?

Yes! Morning sickness can be serious, and we are serious about morning sickness. It's not just in your head, and it can be making you uncomfortable at least, and very ill at worst.

If someone in your life isn't taking you seriously, you are probably understandably upset. Here's what to do.

- *Really relax, such as by doing breathing exercises. (See "MomMy Time" Try Breathing Exercises on page 25.)* •
- *Take some time alone to think about how you feel, maybe even to meditate on it.*
- *Talk it over with a close friend, counselor, or minister.*
- *Write it down in a letter, which you can destroy if you want.*

Once you have sorted out your feelings, talk with the person about how you feel. Use "When. . .I" statements, such as "When you don't listen to me, I feel frustrated."

During my pregnancies, I had a lot of nausea. I tried ginger candy, but it didn't really help. Eating frequent small meals and snacks, especially crackers, helped. Sometimes drinking orange juice helped.

Just goes to show a little trial and error might be worth it to figure out what you can and can't tolerate.

—*Rachel S. Rohde, MD, a mom of a six-year-old daughter and a newborn, an associate professor of orthopaedic surgery at the Oakland University William Beaumont School of Medicine, and an orthopaedic upper extremity surgeon with Michigan Orthopaedic Institute, P.C., in Southfield, MI*

I know a lot of people swear by Coke and ginger ale for nausea, but I've never been a soda drinker.

I never even tried it when I was pregnant. Instead, I drank mainly water.

—*Eva Ritvo, MD*

Morning sickness was tough with my first pregnancy. It started just after the "hit by a train" crushing exhaustion that prompted me to find out I was pregnant.

During my first pregnancy, drinking ice and tea with milk were enough to get me past. I was on rounds and nauseated, but it was more uncomfortable than unbearable.

—*Amy Baxter, MD*

One of the few things that I could drink when my morning sickness was bad was orange Gatorade. I'm very worried that I'm going to fail my glucose tolerance test in a few months because I've been drinking so much sugar!

Eating a balanced diet is especially important during pregnancy. Now I've consciously increased my water intake, and I'm eating more fruits, vegetables, and meat.

—*Michelle Davis-Dash, MD*

When I was battling morning sickness, a friend told me about Sea-Band anti-nausea wristbands. Wearing them didn't provide major relief, like medication might, but they did offer me some benefit by lessening my nausea, with no side effects.

—*Eva Ritvo, MD*

During my second pregnancy, I tried pressing acupressure points in my wrist when it got severe. I pressed on the points with my opposite hand until my nausea subsided. Today you can buy wristbands that do this, such as PsiBands, which keep constant pressure on those points.

—*Amy Baxter, MD*

Ginger for nausea is underrated. When I had morning sickness, I drank ginger tea and flat ginger ale, and I ate ginger candy. Remedies like ginger aren't as risky as the drugs we often throw at people.

—*Susan Wilder, MD*

In my most recent and third pregnancy, my morning sickness really was in the morning—as opposed to my second pregnancy when I felt worse at night. This time my morning sickness was significant, but pretty tame. I only threw up a couple

? When to Call Your Doctor or Midwife

You know that feeling crummy is a small part of pregnancy, but if morning sickness is severe, your doctor may prescribe a medication or recommend taking a supplement. Here's a list of morning sickness symptoms that warrant an immediate phone call to your physician or midwife.

- Vomiting blood or if your vomit looks like coffee grounds, which may be a sign of blood
- Persistent nausea that interferes with your ability to eat and drink throughout the day
- Nausea and vomiting that start *after* nine weeks of pregnancy
- Vomiting three to four times a day and not being able to keep food down
- Weight loss of more than two pounds
- Urinating much less often or much more often than usual
- Abdominal pain or tenderness
- Fever
- Fainting
- Dizziness

of times, which was dramatically better than pregnancy #2.

At the first sign of nausea, I sucked on a Preggie Pop or chewed some ginger gum. That seemed to keep things in check for me.

- Rapid heart rate
- Severe headaches
- Confusion
- Extreme fatigue
- Swelling in the front of your neck, which could be a sign of an enlarged thyroid gland
- Feeling very thirsty and having a dry tongue
- Body odor along with rapid fat loss
- Anxiety or depression

Other symptoms that you should mention at your next doctor or midwife appointment include food aversions; a sensitive gag reflex; trouble sleeping; salivating excessively; a more sensitive sense of smell; changes in your skin so that it's less elastic or it looks pale, dry, or waxy; and sensitivity to noise, light, and motion.

If the nausea and vomiting don't go away after your 16th week of pregnancy, talk with your doctor. This can be normal for some (unfortunate!) women, but it's still a good idea to discuss it with your physician.

My favorite flavors of Preggie Pops were the sour lemon and sour tangerine. These were so yummy, though, that my daughter always snuck one or two for herself.

—Sigrid Payne DaVeiga, MD, a mom of 11-year-old and 6-month-old sons and a 6-year-old daughter and a pediatric allergist with the Children's Hospital of Philadelphia, in Philadelphia, PA

∽

At one point during my second pregnancy, after taking our first family trip to Disney World, I was curled up in a ball in the Orlando airport lounge, unwilling to move because of the nausea. This was part of what prompted me to create the Baxter Animated Retching Faces scale to evaluate pediatric nausea. I realized that you can be extremely nauseated but not throw up. Because most studies of chemo in kids use throwing up as their outcome, they're missing a lot of nausea.

You might use this scale yourself for tracking your own nausea.

—Amy Baxter, MD

∽

I had tremendous morning sickness. It started five weeks into my pregnancy, and it lasted pretty much until my second trimester. Every. Single. Day.

I was sensitive to daylight! Every time I went outside, I would get very nauseated. Sometimes I'd even throw up. I had to wear three pairs of sunglasses, one on top of the other!

—Nilong Parikh Vyas, MD, MPH

During my first pregnancy, I was a medical resident at Cornell. I remember feeling very, very tired. I'd work all day, come home, and take a nap. I'd sleep on the couch until my husband would wake me up and tell me it was late enough to go to bed. It was exhausting. I also had some nausea.

—*Eva Ritvo, MD*

∽

I never had morning sickness, but in my third pregnancy, I had what felt like a delayed afternoon hangover almost every day between 2 pm and 4 pm. It started in my second trimester.

I thought of it as an afternoon slump. I could never associate it with anything other than that I was pregnant and it was the afternoon.

I felt queasy, and my stomach always felt like I was on the verge of retching, but I never did. I would also get a dull headache and feel foggy.

It was very difficult to cope. On really bad days, I would take an anti-nausea medication, such as ondansetron (Zofran). The medicine would help, but, like a hangover, on most days it would just have to get better on its own.

It was very frustrating to have nothing I could take to make me feel better, and the whole time I was still working full-time as an ob-gyn. I gained a new appreciation for my patients with hyperemesis.

—*Marra S. Francis, MD, a mom of 10-, 11-, 13-, and 17-year-old daughters and a 22-year-old son and an ob-gyn, in San Antonio, TX*

When my morning sickness was at its peak, even chewing gum made me sick. The mint flavor was the worst. Toothpaste tasted awful to me. Ironic, right?

I usually don't rinse and spit; I just leave the toothpaste on my teeth. But when my nausea was really bad, I had to rinse.

—*Michelle Davis-Dash, MD*

I think I was lucky. My morning sickness was never terrible. Brushing my teeth was difficult, though.

—*Rebecca Jeanmonod, MD*

In my second pregnancy, I had a very hard time keeping my prenatal vitamins down. In my third pregnancy, I was determined to take them because I was very nervous about the low iron levels I had in my second pregnancy. I found that I could really tolerate the One-A-Day Prenatal vitamin, without the supplemental DHA/ARA portion that is an optional add-on in that vitamin packaging.

—*Sigrid Payne DaVeiga*

Nausea is like chronic pain. It wears you down, and it really sucks the energy and joy out of life. I was so grateful that my morning sickness only lasted for a short time. And when I got to hold my babies in my arms, it all was so worth it!

—*Amy Baxter, MD*

GI PRO TIP: Treat Yourself Gingerly

Ginger is an old-fashioned natural therapy for nausea and vomiting.

Ginger eases many gastrointestinal symptoms, including morning sickness. Ginger is gentle enough to sprinkle on your couscous, but it's also powerful enough to treat nausea in people taking chemotherapy for cancer.

The part of ginger that's effective is the root, which contains two types of plant chemicals that help alleviate nausea and vomiting—gingerols and shogaols. These beneficial substances work directly in the gastrointestinal tract to increase gastric tone and motility, and to speed gastric emptying. When food moves a little faster out of your stomach, there's less time for it to come back up.

Most of the clinical studies on ginger and nausea suggest it's safe to take 1,000 milligrams of ginger each day, even during pregnancy. You can buy ginger in a variety of preparations; 1,000 milligrams, or one gram, is equal to:

1 teaspoon (5 grams) freshly grated ginger

2 milliliters liquid ginger extract

4 cups (235 milliliters each) prepackaged ginger tea

2 teaspoons ginger syrup (10 milliliters)

2 pieces crystallized ginger (each 1 inch long)

You don't have to take the dose all at once. Instead, you can divide it into two or three doses and take them over a 24-hour period.

—*Stacey Ann Weiland, MD*

I think with morning sickness, as with most things, mental attitude plays a part. Most women have heard of morning sickness. If you head into pregnancy convinced that you're going to get morning sickness, you probably will.

On the other hand, if you go into pregnancy confident that you're going to feel well, that the opportunity to build a new body is the greatest gift, and that you'll have few physical symptoms, then that's probably a self-fulfilling prophecy too.

Most women have some morning sickness. I did in my first pregnancy. But if you dwell on it, you'll feel worse. But if you distract yourself and try to think of other things, it will likely get better.

Most women can manage morning sickness. You can look forward to the fact that it usually goes away around week 12. Knowing that something uncomfortable has a time limit helps an awful lot.

—*Eva Ritvo, MD*

I had morning sickness during all three of my pregnancies. Fortunately, for me, the nausea during all three pregnancies seemed to gradually fade away around three months. One day I realized, "Hey! I haven't been nauseated in a few days!"

—*Amy Baxter, MD*

Mommy MD Guides-Recommended Product
Preggie Pops

You never know when morning sickness will hit. It's not always in the a.m.! You can be prepared to ease the symptom by storing Preggie Pops in your purse or in your desk. These naturally flavored, specially formulated, gluten-free lollipops can offer drug-free relief for your queasiness. They contain specific essential oils that are known to soothe your stomach and act as aromatherapy agents. They also contain sugars to work on a queasy stomach caused by hypoglycemia, or low blood sugar. Use them throughout your pregnancy and pack them in your hospital bag. They'll help with dry mouth and give you energy during labor. You'll need it!

A box of seven lollipops In mint, sour fruit, or a variety pack that includes lavender, ginger, mint, and sour fruit costs $3.95. You can buy them in drugstores and at major retailers. For more information, go to **THREELOLLIES.COM.**

In both of my pregnancies, I was very negatively affected by morning sickness. I was so relieved when it abated in my second trimester. It was like a light switch going off.

—*Nilong Parikh Vyas, MD, MPH*

Dr. Jim's Tip
WHERE'S MY VILLAGE?
DOES SOCIAL SUPPORT HELP?

Yes! Studies suggest that it does.

One study of 243 pregnant women in Taiwan found that women who had high levels of stress had more severe morning sickness, but that it could be helped with social support.

Another study of 10 pregnant women in Taiwan found that social support was among the four most important factors in the moms-to-be dealt with nausea and vomiting.

In general, experts say that having supportive family members and friends can help you feel more positive about your health, even when you're feeling sick to your stomach.

Now is the time to reach out to the important people in your life. You may find that surrounding yourself with loving people will help you feel better.

People are probably longing to spend more time with you right now, anxious to hear about your pregnancy and dreams for your future. Perhaps you could invite a friend or family member to breakfast, lunch, or coffee.

Pregnancy is also a great time to reach out to other women. You'll find many actual support groups in your local area and virtual ones online.

GI PRO TIP: Look on the Bright Side

While it can be a major bummer for a newly pregnant woman to have to deal with a constant feeling of nausea and occasional vomiting, one of the biggest boosts I've been able to give my patients is when I inform them that feeling this way is actually a sign of a healthy pregnancy!

Data from the Norwegian Mother and Child Cohort Study (MoBa), which followed more than 50,000 pregnancies from 1999 to 2008, found that women who had morning sickness tended to have better delivery and birth outcomes compared with moms who didn't have morning sickness. Babies born to moms with morning sickness had a lower chance of requiring emergency C-section delivery, and they had *higher* Apgar scores (which are tests given to assess a baby's health immediately after birth) and birth weights.

Here's another interesting side note: Moms who had morning sickness were more likely to have girls.

—Stacey Ann Weiland, MD

Never underestimate the importance of social support. It's important to our well-being and to our longevity. We know that people with cancer who have social support live longer. People going through divorce with social support do better.

I don't know of any research about the effect of social support on pregnancy and morning sickness, but it makes sense that if you feel supported, you feel better. When you get a hug, your body secretes oxytocin, which is nature's bonding hormone. It makes you feel relaxed, content, connected, good!

A mom-to-be who's supported will have an easier time in pregnancy than a mom-to-be who feels alone. If you have help, you worry less about things. If you worry less, you'll have less stress. If you feel less stress, your body will produce less cortisol. And you'll feel better!

There are many ways to find support during pregnancy. It's wonderful, of course, if you have a supportive marital partner. But you might also have extra family support and really good friends. Even connecting with people on social media can help.

Back when our ancestors were hunter-gatherers, they lived in groups of about 150 people. Everyone supported and helped everyone else. For the past few generations, we have lived isolated lives, largely with just our own families. Today with social media, our network—our world—has greatly expanded once again.

When I was pregnant for the first time, I was completing my medical residency. Nine of us residents got pregnant and gave birth around the same time! We used to joke that there was something in the water. We felt very supported and protected. It was a very exciting time. I felt like I was doing the right thing, at the right time—engaging in the rhythm of life.

—*Eva Ritvo, MD*

YouTube Funny Videos

It's impossible not to smile at the sight and sound of a giggling baby, a gurgling baby, a surprised baby, or even a messy baby. (Get ready!) The categories of funny baby videos online are endless (babies trying new foods, babies at the zoo, babies with pets, babies seeing their reflections...), and they can offer a distraction to your pesky pregnancy symptoms.

Funny videos can also be a reminder of why your morning sickness will all be worth it. You may even find inspiration to record your own cute baby videos once your little one arrives.

When I was struggling with morning sickness, I followed the same advice I tell my post-op anesthesia/surgical patients who might experience post-op nausea and vomiting. I made sure I stayed hydrated by drinking water, and as long as I was urinating, I wasn't too concerned. When the nausea passed, I usually started off eating something bland, such as toast, and progressed from there. Every day my symptoms improved, and by the second trimester I was craving Taco Bell!

—Edna Ma, MD, a mom of a 4-year-old son and an 18-month-old daughter, an anesthesiologist, and the founder of BareEASE pre-waxing numbing kit, in Los Angeles, CA

My nausea was really awful at times. Sometimes I feared my whole pregnancy would be like this. You just kind of have to hold on and keep the faith that it will get better.

Whatever you do, don't Google! It always shows you the worst side of everything.

Instead, listen to your body. Do what your body tells you to do. And hang on and enjoy the ride.

—*Michelle Davis-Dash, MD*

Dr. Rallie's Tip

My husband and I aren't highly organized humans, so we didn't exactly plan our pregnancies, which explains why we had two babies in two years! We just knew we were ready for our children, and we'd welcome them whenever they arrived, even if it was back-to-back.

Because I wasn't expecting to be expecting, morning sickness was always the first sign that I was pregnant. It usually struck for the first time at around six weeks of pregnancy, first thing in the morning.

For me, morning sickness lasted right through the first trimester. In those early weeks of pregnancy, I could count on waking up and feeling sick for 15 minutes to a half hour every morning. Sometimes I'd actually throw up, which was a blessed relief because it made me feel better right away, and I could move forward with my day.

Other times I would just gag, which was miserable.

Sometimes when it was really bad, I would sit on the edge of the tub next to my buddy the toilet bowl until the feeling passed.

For the second half of my first trimester of pregnancy, dealing with morning sickness was a very big part of my morning routine.

I learned not to brush my teeth until the nausea had passed. A toothbrush can stimulate your gag reflex like nothing else. I also learned that if I took my prenatal vitamins when I was feeling the slightest bit nauseated, I was sure to throw up. So I started to take my prenatal vitamin in the evening, once my stomach was fully settled.

The best thing about my morning sickness was that it usually occurred as soon as I woke up, regardless of the time. I could wake up at 6 am or 8:30 am, and either way I'd be sick. Once I discovered this, I simply started setting my alarm clock to go off an hour earlier to give myself time to get past the nausea so I wouldn't be late for work.

I tried keeping crackers on my nightstand and eating one or two or 10 before I climbed out of bed, but that didn't work for me. I was going to feel sick—or be sick!—one way or another. The thing that worked best for me was just giving myself an extra hour in my morning routine before I started the whole shower-hair-makeup business. It's hard to put on mascara with your head hovering over the toilet.

When I was feeling sick, I really tried not to feel sorry for myself. Most of us associate feelings of nausea and throwing up with illness, and this can be a little depressing. It's important to remember that morning sickness is often part of a healthy, thriving pregnancy, so don't let it get you down. When I was feeling sick, I tried to conjure up positive thoughts, like "Thank heavens my hormones are so potent!" and "Morning sickness is surely a sign of a healthy pregnancy!"

I also tried not to feel resentment toward my husband, who was usually snoozing blissfully in bed while I was camped out by the commode. I didn't work very hard at that.

Once the wave or waves of nausea passed, I was usually fine for the rest of the day. I could leave my post by the potty, take a shower, eat a nutritious breakfast, and feel perfectly normal, like it never even happened. I think that giving myself extra time in the mornings to deal with morning sickness really helped. That way I didn't feel rushed or overwhelmed, and I didn't worry that I was going to be late for work, which only made me feel worse.

When all else fails, remember that morning sickness doesn't last forever. One day you'll wake up and poof, it'll be gone!

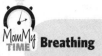

Breathing

It's amazing that something as simple as breathing can calm you down and ease your worries. But it's true: Regular, mindful breathing can help reduce stress and paradoxically give you energy. Here's one breathing technique that you can use twice a day, or even just when you find your mind swelling on upsetting thoughts.

Sit in a comfortable chair. Place your right hand on your chest and your left hand on your abdomen. Take a deep breath in through your nose. You should notice that your hand on your abdomen is rising higher than your hand on your chest. Slowly exhale through your mouth. Next, take a slow, deep breath in through your nose. Hold it for a count of seven. Slowly exhale through your mouth for a count of eight.

Gently contract your ab muscles to completely get all of the air out of your lungs. This is the key to exercise: Exhaling all of the air out of your body. Repeat the cycle four more times. Once you have this pattern down, you might want to add words to make it work even better. For example, when you inhale, you could say to yourself the feeling that you want to have, such as "relaxation," and when you exhale, you could say to yourself the feeling that you want to get rid of, such as "stress."

Chapter 2

Ptyalism

Welcome to the world of motherhood, which is filled with things that no one ever tells you about! Ever heard of ptyalism? Most moms-to-be haven't. Yet many women develop it early in pregnancy along with morning sickness.

Ptyalism is also called excess salivation or hypersalivation. If you develop this condition, you might feel like you have too much saliva in your mouth, or like you can't swallow all of the spit in your mouth. You might have a bad taste in your mouth, and your saliva might seem too thick.

It's usually only bothersome during the day, but for some women, it wakes them up during the night.

This feeling of too much saliva is unlike any feeling outside of pregnancy. It can be uncomfortable, annoying, and downright distressing.

The good news is, ptyalism usually goes away along with your first trimester. For some women, however, it gets worse, and they have it throughout their pregnancies.

Similar to morning sickness, no one knows what causes ptyalism. (Are you sensing a theme here?) Researchers think that ptyalism occurs because the parasympathetic nerves of the salivary glands are stimulated by pregnancy, causing a profuse watery secretion—too much spit.

Justification for a Celebration
No longer needing to spit into a cup will be cause to celebrate!

With this pregnancy, in addition to my severe morning sickness, I have too much spit in my mouth, and my spit feels too thick. It's horrendous!

I can't swallow all of this saliva. I have to spit it out. I keep handkerchiefs stashed everywhere—in my lab coat pockets, in my car, in my office.

I force myself to drink water. That helps a little bit.

—Michelle Davis-Dash, MD, a mom of a 5-year-old son, who's expecting another baby, and a pediatrician in Baltimore, MD

When to Call Your Doctor or Midwife

Ptyalism, which is characterized by excessive saliva, is often a sign of severe morning sickness. It's usually accompanied by excessive nausea and vomiting.

Be sure to call your doctor if you're experiencing this condition and if you're having extreme nausea or any other worrisome symptoms, such as vomiting several times a day, not being able to eat or drink, losing more than two pounds of weight, and other symptoms listed in "When to Call Your Doctor or Midwife" on page 10.

If you ever vomit blood or a substance that looks like coffee grounds, get immediate medical attention.

> **If I spit, they will take my spit
> and frame it like a work of art.**
>
> —*Pablo Picasso*

When I was pregnant, my mouth would fill up with saliva whenever I brushed my teeth. It's called hypersalivation, or ptyalism. Sometimes we see this in children, too, when they're nauseated. Their salivary glands make too much saliva.

There's not too much to do about it. I just swallowed a lot.

—*Rebecca Jeanmonod, MD, a mom of 12- and 8-year-old daughters and 11- and 8-year-old sons and a professor of emergency medicine and the associate residency program director for the emergency medicine residency at St. Luke's University Health Network, in Bethlehem, PA*

⁓

I had very mild morning sickness; really it was all day sickness. My symptom was a sour taste in my mouth as if I were about to vomit all day. My Ob said that it was a form or morning sickness. I chewed gum and ate very spicy food to distract myself.

—*Dina Strachan, MD, a mom of one eight-year-old daughter, a dermatologist and director of Aglow Dermatology, and an assistant clinical professor in the department of dermatology at New York University in New York City*

GI PRO TIP: Spit Less

Ptyalism gravidarum, or excess saliva production, during pregnancy can be a distressing and uncomfortable condition. Often associated with morning sickness, nausea, and hyperemesis gravidarum, ptyalism generally occurs in the absence of any salivary gland disease. Because it so often occurs together with nausea and vomiting, ptyalism often goes away with anti-nausea treatments.

Here are some tips to try.

- Eat smaller, more frequent meals.
- Brush your teeth and use mouthwash several times per day.
- Chew sugarless gum.
- Suck on hard candies or mints. (Occupying your mouth with sweet and minty flavors won't stop saliva production, but it will make your mouth feel fresher and cleaner.)
- Take frequent, small sips of water.
- Avoid smoking. (Smoking increases saliva production, which is yet another reason to quit!)
- Talk to your dentist about gum disease or other mouth problems. (Tooth and gum problems can arise during pregnancy too!)
- Avoid high-carb, high-starch foods, such as potatoes.
- Suck on ice cubes or ice pops. (They make your mouth feel numb and reduce saliva production.)
- Suck on a lime or piece of ginger.

—Stacey Ann Weiland, MD

Buy Yourself Flowers

Here's a way to treat yourself and help to alleviate nausea: Buy a beautiful bouquet of flowers with tummy-calming scents, such as lavender or mint. Breathing in these scents might help your gastrointestinal tract to stop the spasms and help you feel less nauseated.

DR. RALLIE'S TIP

I was very fortunate not to have ptyalism, but during the morning sickness phase of each pregnancy, I did experience the temporary gush of saliva that often accompanies nausea. It was such a miserable feeling. I tried to focus on being thankful that it lasted for only an hour or so. Pregnancy is not for weaklings. This is nine months of hard, challenging work, and it's not all ponies and rainbows. At times, some of the conditions that accompany pregnancy seem almost unbearable. I suppose it's Nature's way of preparing us for motherhood. In a few short months, when you're gazing into the eyes of your amazing, precious newborn and experiencing the deepest love imaginable, you'll be struck by the realization that you would gladly walk through fire for this tiny person. If you're suffering from one of pregnancy's more intolerable or insulting maladies, whether it's ptyalism or giant hemorrhoids or raging heartburn, you can console yourself with the knowledge that you're just paying it forward.

GI PRO TIP
Feel Very Sleepy...

Hypnosis can be helpful for pregnant women with ptyalism. Approved by the American Medical Association as a legitimate medical treatment since 1958, hypnosis has been used to help pregnant women cope with the pain of labor and to ease the symptoms of hyperemesis gravidarum.

In a case report published in the *American Journal of Clinical Hypnosis* in 2015, a 28-year-old woman was successfully treated for ptyalism and hyperemesis gravidarum with weekly hypnosis sessions from week 16 to week 36 of pregnancy.

Hypnosis may work to reduce ptyalism in several ways. First, hypnosis places a patient in a deep state of physiologic relaxation, which reduces the activity of the sympathetic nervous system. In addition, during a hypnosis session, the hypnotist can give the patient both indirect and direct suggestions that help relax the muscles of the mouth, throat, and stomach. By using muscle tension as a hypnotic cue, the patient may be trained to alternatively engage in pleasant imagery or hold thoughts that mentally reframe the experience to cause the unpleasant symptoms to subside.

—*Stacey Ann Weiland, MD*

DR. JIM'S TIP
DOES MORNING SICKNESS
MAKE FOR SMARTER BABIES?

Maybe! A study published in the Journal of Pediatrics *asked 121 mothers during phone interviews about their morning sickness symptoms and whether or not they took an anti-nausea medication during their pregnancy. The researchers followed up when the children were ages three to seven by giving the mothers IQ tests.*

They found that the mothers who experienced morning sickness had children who tested with higher IQs and scored better when it came to fluency, speech sounds, and numerical memory.

Your takeaway? Take comfort in the thought that you're growing a smart, healthy baby!

Capitalize on this by taking time each day to read and sing to your growing baby. She hears every word you say! When she's born, she will recognize and respond to your loving voice immediately.

Mommy MD Guides–Recommended Product
Preggie Pop Drops

Get rid of a queasy stomach—and that feeling of having too much spit—with Preggie Pop Drops. You'll get all of the benefits from Preggie Pop lollipops, but in a convenient, individually wrapped lozenge.

A container of 21 drops costs $5.50 and comes in sour fruit and green apple flavors. Find them in drugstores, retail stores, or at THREELOLLIES.COM.

Preggie Drops also come in organic varieties. These drops are made with organic evaporated cane juice, organic brown rice syrup, citric acid, and natural flavors and colors. A box of 12 natural lozenges costs $4.95.

If you like the flavor of ginger, consider Preggie Pops Drops Ginger with Brown Rice. Studies have shown that ginger is more effective than a placebo at relieving morning sickness. A container of 21 costs $4.95.

You might also consider Preggie Naturals. These chewy treats are made with brown rice, and they contain 10 milligrams of vitamin B_6. Flavors include ginger, raspberry, or a variety pack with peppermint, raspberry, ginger, and green apple flavors. A box of 15 costs $3.95.

Chapter 3

Sensitivity to Smells and Tastes

Heightened smell sensitivity, which is called hyperosmia, in pregnancy is a real phenomenon. It's not your imagination! It happens usually during the first trimester of pregnancy.

There might be a very good evolutionary reason for why you're not loving the smell of coffee in the morning! Our female ancestors might have evolved to develop hyperosmia during pregnancy to prevent them from eating poisonous substances that could have harmed them or their developing babies.

Hyperosmia is likely related to hormonal changes, and it seems to increase right along with the level of hCG, which is the hormone the body makes during pregnancy. Estrogen may play a role as well. Studies in pregnant mice demonstrated the growth of nerve cells in the vomeronasal organ (VNO), which is a component of the olfactory system located within the lower nose.

Fortunately, your super sniffer will probably settle down as your pregnancy progresses. Unfortunately, a big reason why your nose will no longer be sensitive is because it will be stuffed up.

Justification for a Celebration

Sometime in the coming weeks, the smells that make you gag right now will smell great to you again. And the foods will *taste* even better!

When I was pregnant, smells really bothered me, especially the smells of fish and chicken. I just had to avoid it as much as possible. The smells of citrus or mint could usually overpower anything that made me feel sick. I kept essential oils or gum in my pocket, and that helped.

—Rachel S. Rohde, MD, a mom of a six-year-old daughter and a newborn, an associate professor of orthopaedic surgery at the Oakland University William Beaumont School of Medicine, and an orthopaedic upper extremity surgeon with Michigan Orthopaedic Institute, P.C., in Southfield, MI

When to Call Your Doctor or Midwife

It's bad enough that pregnancy can give you a stronger gag reflex. When Mother Nature turns up your olfactory sense, it can make nausea and vomiting even worse.

One study found that pregnant women with greater smell sensitivity had more severe nausea and vomiting. However, other studies haven't found a clear correlation between the two.

If your increased sensitivity to smell is contributing to severe nausea and vomiting and you're experiencing any of the red flag signs (see "When to Call Your Doctor or Midwife" on page 10), be sure to call your obstetrician or midwife.

When I was pregnant, I couldn't tolerate certain smells—like pizza.

As luck would have it, I had to pass a pizza place on my way into work, through the mall to the metro station. I just couldn't deal with it! I had to bypass that mall.

—*Susan Wilder, MD, a mom of a 22-year-old daughter and twin 17-year-old girls, a primary care physician, and the founder and CEO of LifeScape Premier LLC, in Scottsdale, AZ*

∾

I had morning sickness with all three of my pregnancies, and each time it was a different experience. With my first pregnancy, my symptoms were fairly mild—except I couldn't smell fish or onions without feeling really sick to my stomach.

One evening, my husband and I were eating at a Mexican restaurant. I remember he ordered a ceviche dish. I was so upset with him for ordering it I ran to the car crying that I had to go home, even though I had normally loved that meal!

—*Sigrid Payne DaVeiga, MD, a mom of 11-year-old and 6-month-old sons and a 6-year-old daughter and a pediatric allergist with the Children's Hospital of Philadelphia, in Philadelphia, PA*

∾

I have a big nose, so I'm generally hypersensitive to smells. During pregnancy, smells haven't made me any more nauseated, but they haven't made me any *less* nauseated either!

I think pregnancy has made my sense of smell more

acute. My house smells funny to me all of the time! My husband has to clean the sink and take out the garbage because if I did it, I would get sick. Plus, I don't have the energy to do it.

I've been relying on my husband a lot to help out with the housework. My house is ridiculously messy right now.

—*Michelle Davis-Dash, MD, a mom of a five-year-old son, who's expecting another baby, and a pediatrician in Baltimore, MD*

Mommy MD Guides–Recommended Product
Sea-Band Antinausea Bands

One of the many challenges of pregnancy is that you can't take many medications while pregnant. Luckily, there's one simple solution for morning sickness that's completely drug free: acupressure. Pressing on the acupressure points on your wrists, called the nei kuan points, often helps alleviate nausea, whether it's caused by morning sickness or a bumpy car ride. You'll find several products on the market that stimulate these points, and one is Sea-Band Antinausea Bands. These elastic wrist bands have plastic studs that apply gentle pressure to the acupressure points. You can buy them online at **SEA-BAND.COM** or in all pharmacies and drugstores.

> A book has got smell. A new book smells great.
> An old book smells even better.
> An old book smells like ancient Egypt.
>
> —*Ray Bradbury*

DR. JIM'S TIP
DO MEN GET MORNING SICKNESS?

Yes! It even has a name: Male morning sickness is called couvade syndrome. The term comes from the French word "couver," which means to brood or to hatch.

Men who experience it may gain weight, see changes in their appetite, and have gastrointestinal problems during their partner's pregnancy. Typically, the symptoms stop after the baby is born.

In one study of 143 soon-to-be dads in Poland, the researchers found men reported symptoms of morning sickness, including changes in their appetite, weight gain, and gas.

If your partner shows signs of morning sickness, it might mean he's empathetic and connecting with you in a very personal way. The researchers of the study said men who are sensitive may take on their partner's symptoms.

What to do? On one hand, you might feel frustrated if your partner is complaining of morning sickness! But it might be more positive to consider him as an ally, a support, even a kindred spirit.

Very early in my pregnancy, I became sensitive to smells.

During my first pregnancy, my husband and I traveled to Patagonia. They eat a fish-based diet. I'm a pescatarian; I eat only fruits, vegetables, and fish. While I was in Patagonia, though, I developed an aversion to salmon. I couldn't stand the smell of it.

During my second pregnancy, I couldn't stand the smell of infant formula. This was a problem because my daughter still needed to drink formula! I wished at the time I had an aversion to the smell of diapers. I didn't have any trouble changing my baby's diapers, but my husband had to mix up the bottles.

—*Rebecca Jeanmonod, MD, a mom of 12- and 8-year-old daughters and 11- and 8-year-old sons and a professor of emergency medicine and the associate residency program director for the emergency medicine residency at St. Luke's University Health Network, in Bethlehem, PA*

During pregnancy, I developed an aversion to certain foods, and it persisted for years after my babies were born.

In my first pregnancy, I was a medical resident. I was working odd hours—and a lot of them, up to 140 hours a week. I had to eat quick and easy foods. I used to eat Pop-Tarts, but sometime during the pregnancy I could no longer stand to eat them. To this day, I still can't.

—*Rebecca Jeanmonod, MD*

When I was pregnant, I was completing my medical residency. Several of my co-residents were also pregnant.

One of them, who was also a friend of mine, really struggled with morning sickness. She took half of a lemon, covered it in linen, carried it around with her, and smelled it when she felt nauseated.

GI PRO TIP: Trust Your Nose

If your nose has gotten a little out of control, here are some ways to rein it in.

- Avoid scents that bother you.
- Don't cook or eat foods that have bothersome smells.
- Have someone else do the cooking. (Is that a cheer we hear!?)
- Leave windows open and consider using a fan to blow in fresh air.
- Wash your clothes more often than usual.
- Use unscented toiletries, deodorant, and cleansers.
- Speak with coworkers, friends, and family members about fragrances and air fresheners that may bother you.
- Avoid smokers. (As if you needed another reason to do this.)
- Sip ginger ale.

I was tempted to try that trick too. But I didn't want us to look like two crazy psychiatrists. I just used my lemon at home.

—*Eva Ritvo, MD, a mom of 25- and 21-year-old daughters, a psychiatrist, and the founder of bekindr.com, a movement to bring more kindness to the world, using neuroscience as the foundation, in Miami Beach, FL*

- Surround yourself with mint, lemon, ginger, citrus, cinnamon, or other scents that you like.
- Consider plug-in air fresheners or scented candles.
- Keep garbage cans empty.
- If the smell of fish bothers you, consider taking a DHA supplement instead.
- Try eating something salty, such as saltines or pretzels.
- Clean out your refrigerator. (Better yet, have someone else clean out your refrigerator!)
- Place a box of baking soda in the refrigerator.
- Seal strong smelling foods in airtight glass lidded containers.
- Keep a pleasant smelling lip balm or a tissue soaked with a pleasant fragrance in your pocket or purse to hold under your nose if you are confronted with an unpleasant odor while out and about.

—Stacey Ann Weiland, MD

Because of my severe morning sickness, I was very sensitive to smells. I couldn't even walk into the hospital cafeteria. The smell made me vomit. Every time.

I was in my residency at the time, and my residency-mates went to the cafeteria and brought food back for me.

Do Pregnancy-Safe Yoga Poses

If morning sickness has you feeling anxious and stressed, yoga can help. Prenatal yoga helps ease anxiety, and it also helps you prepare for childbirth. Yoga can make delivery less painful and may even improve the health of your baby.

Choose prenatal yoga, hatha yoga, or restorative yoga during pregnancy. You'll be able to practice breathing techniques, do gentle stretching, and get into yoga postures appropriate for pregnancy. Avoid bikram yoga, which is also called hot yoga, because it will elevate your body temperature, which isn't good for your baby.

For safety, be sure to talk to your doctor before starting a yoga program. Once you start your program, don't overdo it, stay cool, and drink plenty of water. Also, don't do deep forward or backward bends during pregnancy. It's also wise to avoid poses in which you twist and put pressure on your belly. Inverted poses are also a no-no. Pregnancy can affect your balance, and you certainly don't want to fall on your head!

My sense of smell was so acute that I couldn't stand the smell of food cooking. My husband cooked outside, on the grill, in the winter, in Iowa, in the snow.

—*Carrie Brown, MD, a mom of 12- and 10-year-old sons and a general pediatrician who treats medically complex children and specializes in palliative care at Arkansas Children's Hospital, in Little Rock*

In my first pregnancy, if I smelled, saw, or even heard the word "ham," I immediately started to choke, gag, and retch. I would have the instant increase in salivary production that happens just before you are about to throw up. It was awful. A few times, I couldn't get away from the source fast enough, and I vomited.

My ham aversion started early in my first trimester. It lasted the entire pregnancy and even for the first few months postpartum. It wasn't until around a year later that I finally tried to eat ham again.

My aversion to the smell of ham was awful for me, but it was a source of great amusement for my friends and family. Sometimes they would look at me and just say the word "ham" to watch me start to gag and run.

I avoided people eating ham sandwiches, never drove by any HoneyBaked Ham storefronts, and asked everyone to please *not* serve ham at any gatherings I planned to attend.

—*Marra S. Francis, MD, a mom of 10-, 11-, 13-, and 17-year-old daughters and a 22-year-old son and an ob-gyn, in San Antonio, TX*

DR. RALLIE'S TIP

During my pregnancy, I wasn't sensitive to most of the familiar smells at home, but the minute I stepped into the hospital, I would begin to feel queasy. I was especially sensitive to chemical odors, including industrial cleaning solutions, air fresheners, and antiseptic soaps and lotions. As soon as I caught a sniff of one of those things, I'd start to feel sick to my stomach.

To counteract the unpleasant, nausea-inducing smells, I carried a small tube of eucalyptus ointment in my pocket. I dabbed a bit of the ointment under my nose whenever the need arose. I found the smell of the eucalyptus blocked the unpleasant odors around me, quelled my nausea, and had a calming effect on me.

I was in my residency training during my second and third pregnancies. I was also plagued with dizziness, especially whenever I had to stand for long periods of time or when I smelled strong odors. Working in the hospital, I was on my feet most of the day, and strong odors were impossible to avoid. Whenever I felt myself getting dizzy, I just had to stop and drop. I'd sit on a chair if I could find one, or I'd plop down on the floor if I couldn't. If I didn't sit down and put my head on my knees, I was sure to faint.

> **For the sense of smell, almost more than any other, has the power to recall memories and it is a pity that we use it so little.**
>
> **—Rachel Carson**

> **You're only here for a short visit.**
> **Don't hurry, don't worry. And be sure**
> **to smell the flowers along the way.**
>
> *—Walter Hagen*

During my pregnancy, I had some odor sensitivity. I avoided strong odors, such as onions, garlic, perfume, and smoke. I also chewed mint gum to try to neutralize the offensive odors. Fresh air really helped; just going outside would make me feel better.

—Jennifer A. Gardner, MD, a mom of seven-year-old son, a pediatrician, and the founder of an online child wellness and weight management company, HealthyKidsCompany.com, in Washington, DC

During my pregnancies, my sense of smell was very heightened. Fortunately, it didn't make me sick. That was a very good thing because I was working in pediatrics at the time, and the diaper smells could have really upset my stomach.

—Eva Mayer, MD, a mom of a 12-year-old daughter and an 11-year-old son, an associate professor of pediatrics at Temple University, and a pediatrician with St. Luke's Pediatrics Associates, in Bethlehem, PA

Chapter 4

Vomiting and Hyperemesis Gravidarum

If you have tried our other tips and tricks for morning sickness and still cannot keep any food down, you may have a more serious condition than morning sickness. While nausea from morning sickness is a pretty common annoyance in pregnancy, a much more serious condition known as hyperemesis gravidarum (HG) will require medical treatment.

Some signs that it is time to call your healthcare professional for help and advice are the inability to keep any food down at all, losing weight, not urinating as often, confusion, low blood pressure, or fainting. Follow your instincts.

It's important not to become dehydrated. Most cases of HG resolve in the first five months of pregnancy and can be treated by administering IV fluids and following the same dietary tips for morning sickness. And, yes, you can still use your Preggie Pops.

JUSTIFICATION FOR A CELEBRATION
The day you stop throwing up—even if it's your baby's birthday—will be a wonderful day to celebrate.

I had some morning sickness during my pregnancies. It wasn't terribly bad. What was challenging was the suddenness of the vomiting. It came completely out of the blue!

One day during my first pregnancy, I was walking my dog, and all of a sudden, I stopped to vomit. My pug looked around at me, and I swear he was thinking, *What the heck?*

It was like in the movie *Fargo*. The cop is pregnant, and she would just stop what she was doing and throw up. That was hysterical—and so true to life.

—*Susan Wilder, MD, a mom of a 22-year-old daughter and twin 17-year-old girls, a primary care physician, and the founder and CEO of LifeScape Premier LLC, in Scottsdale, AZ*

During my pregnancies, I had a lot of nausea up until week 16. During my first pregnancy, my nausea was so bad. My doctor prescribed ondansetron (Zofran), which blocks the actions of chemicals in the body that can trigger nausea and vomiting.

Unfortunately, just when the morning sickness kicked in during my second pregnancy, Zofran had been pulled off of the "safe during pregnancy" list.

I tried taking the combination of over-the-counter Unisom and vitamin B_6, which physicians joke is the "poor man's Diclegis." That did nothing for me—except make me sleepy.

Fortunately, I only had a few episodes of vomiting. I just suffered through them and hoped it would pass soon.

—Rachel S. Rohde, MD, a mom of a six-year-old daughter and a newborn, an associate professor of orthopaedic surgery at the Oakland University William Beaumont School of Medicine, and an orthopaedic upper extremity surgeon with Michigan Orthopaedic Institute, P.C., in Southfield, MI

∽

I threw up only once during pregnancy. It was right after I took one of those huge prenatal vitamins. It got stuck in my throat and made me throw up.

—Eva Ritvo, MD, a mom of 25- and 21-year-old daughters, a psychiatrist, and the founder of bekindr.com, a movement to bring more kindness to the world, using neuroscience as the foundation, in Miami Beach, FL.

DR. JIM'S TIP
CAN YOU BLAME YOUR MOM?

Maybe!

Morning sickness might have both a hereditary and cultural basis.

One study found that moms-to-be whose sisters had severe morning sickness, HG, were a whopping 17 times more likely to also develop HG. An earlier study, of twins, also found that if one twin had morning sickness, the other was more likely to as well.

In this pregnancy, I've thrown up so much that there's nothing left in my stomach. I vomit foam.

I have to force myself to drink so I don't get dehydrated. The least awful things to drink are orange Gatorade and ginger ale. But it's pretty much an endless cycle: I force myself to drink, and then I throw up.

When to Call Your Doctor or Midwife

If you're experiencing vomiting that goes beyond typical morning sickness—your nausea doesn't go away, you vomit several times a day, you have lost your appetite, you're dehydrated (signs include infrequent urination and extreme thirst), you feel faint, or you've experienced weight loss of more than two pounds—don't delay calling your doctor.

When nausea and vomiting are severe, you might need medication or even hospitalization to replace fluids and nutrients. Your doctor may also want to be sure vomiting isn't related to an illness, such as a urinary tract infection. Also, remember to call your doctor without delay if you vomit blood or your vomit resembles coffee grounds, which can be a sign of blood.

While morning sickness in early pregnancy and occasional vomiting later on are usually benign, sometimes nausea and vomiting can indicate more serious medical

It was very difficult with HG to drink any sort of liquid. There's a real risk for dehydration.

conditions. Any of the following signs or symptoms warrant a call to your doctor or midwife.

- Fever or chills
- Persistent abdominal pain
- Abdominal pain radiating to your back
- Colicky abdominal pain (pain that comes and goes)
- Vaginal bleeding, or a change in vaginal discharge
- Vomiting blood or "coffee ground" material
- Blood in the stool or black stool
- Blood in the urine and/or painful urination
- Yellowing of the skin or the whites of the eyes
- Visual disturbances
- Severe headache
- Severe swelling of the hands, legs, or face
- Light-headedness

I forced myself to drink as much as I could, and I could usually drink Sprite and Gatorade. Twice I got so dehydrated that I had to go to the hospital to get IV fluids.

—*Carrie Brown, MD, a mom of 12- and 10-year-old sons and a general pediatrician who treats medically complex children and specializes in palliative care at Arkansas Children's Hospital, in Little Rock*

My morning sickness has been so terrible in this pregnancy that I have to force myself to eat. I did lose a few pounds, but at my nine-week ultrasound the baby was fine, so that eased my mind.

Even though I know I'm likely to throw up food, I make myself eat anyway. Some foods I can eat are crackers, fruit, and baked or roasted chicken.

I can will myself to eat, but it's usually inevitable that I'll throw it back up. Sometimes mind-over-matter can get you only so far!

—*Michelle Davis-Dash, MD*

Eating with severe morning sickness was very difficult for me. Anytime I thought I might possibly be able to eat something and keep it down, my husband would get it for me. Even if that meant he was roused from a deep sleep to get out of bed and go through a drive-thru in his pajamas, he did it.

One night, I thought I could eat a Big Mac. My husband

said, "I'll be right back." Ten minutes later, he came back dripping wet. He didn't complain even once that it was pouring rain outside!

Sometimes whatever I was craving would stay down; other times it would come back up. There was simply no way to tell.

I'm not a skinny person. I lost 30 to 40 pounds in my first pregnancy. Thank goodness, my son was fine. My obstetrician used to joke that I was "living off of the fat of the land." I didn't find that funny when I was pregnant, but I can find humor in it now!

—*Carrie Brown, MD*

∽◦◦

In my third pregnancy, with my twins, my biggest problem occurred when I ate too late in the day. Inevitably, it would come back up after I went to bed. I had to stop eating solid food in the afternoon.

I gained 75 pounds during that pregnancy. The pressure in my stomach was so great that it felt like there was no room for food.

I drank a lot of juice and tea. I could also drink just about anything that melted, like ice cream.

—*Rebecca Jeanmonod, MD, a mom of 12- and 8-year-old daughters and 11- and 8-year-old sons and a professor of emergency medicine and the associate residency program director for the emergency medicine residency at St. Luke's University Health Network, in Bethlehem, PA*

In my first pregnancy, I was in my medical residency, and I needed to limit the time I spent throwing up. Emergency medicine is a very male-dominated field. There's a lot of prejudice against women physicians getting pregnant. Even today, in job interviews, they'll hint, "Hopefully you're done with babies." It's not legal, or right, but it happens.

In the residency program where I teach, three female physicians gave birth last year. The only pregnant woman we

When to Call Your Doctor or Midwife

For expectant moms, severe or constant morning sickness might seem to be hyperemesis gravidarum (HG). HG develops over time, so especially early in your pregnancy, it may be difficult to know if you have it.

And while some severe cases of morning sickness *do* progress to HG if not effectively treated, there are ways to distinguish between the two. In general, the classic signs and symptoms of HG are:

- Severe nausea and vomiting
- Rapid weight loss of one to two pounds a week (or more)
- Weight loss greater than 5 percent of your pre-pregnancy weight
- Recurrent dehydration and electrolyte imbalance

didn't hear discussion about was the one who took only two weeks off to have her baby. The male residents have lots of babies, but because they don't need to take time off, no one gives them grief. But they're not physically birthing a child.

My doctor prescribed Ridlan. It's a class B anti-nausea medication, which means you can take it during pregnancy. It promotes gut motility, so it helps prevent vomiting. It helps move food out of your stomach before you can throw it up.

—*Rebecca Jeanmonod, MD*

Talking with your doctor or midwife is vital in treating HG. A number of medications have been used for many years, and they pose little risk to your unborn baby, even if they're taken early in pregnancy. In many cases, the risks of HG are greater than the risks of taking the medications.

Call your doctor or midwife if you:

- Cannot keep more than a few bites of food or a few sips of water down for 24 hours or more
- Lose two or more pounds in one week
- Vomit blood
- Faint or generally feel very ill

Finally, remember that if you feel weak or dizzy, you'll definitely need someone to take you to the emergency department.

When I was severely sick, I just did as much as I could. I wasn't diagnosed with HG; it never got to that point. I didn't meet the criteria for HG: My blood pressure stayed the same, and I didn't lose that much weight. It was just very bad morning sickness.

I prayed that it didn't progress to HG, and I was so grateful that it didn't.

—*Michelle Davis-Dash, MD*

Even though my morning sickness was severe, I still had to work. If I needed to throw up, I raced to a bathroom.

I work in a medical group, and my coworkers are terrific. They really look out for me. They make sure we have plenty of orange Gatorade at the office. That's one of the few things I can consistently keep down.

I was lucky that at the time my sickness was the worst, it was summer, which is a slower time for our medical practice. I wasn't as busy as I might have been a few months back. My workload was doable.

When I get very tired at work, I take a nap in my office. I keep a few extra lab coats in my office to snuggle under. I have an exam table and a couch in there. I sleep on the couch because I worry I'll roll right off the exam table onto the floor.

—*Michelle Davis-Dash, MD*

At one point during this pregnancy, I had to go on a car trip. My husband, our son, and I drove 9 ½ hours from Baltimore, MD,

> **Calling HG morning sickness
> is like calling a hurricane a little rain.**
>
> —*Anonymous*

to Columbia, SC, to attend a wedding.

I'm a mind-over-matter person, so I tried to convince myself it would be okay. That didn't work.

I kept having to ask my husband to pull off the highway at rest stops so that I could throw up. I blamed my need to stop on my son. I said that he had to use the bathroom.

"But I don't *have to go* to the bathroom," my son would say.

"Oh, yes, you do!" I'd reply.

When I knew I had to throw up, I could keep it down as long as I knew my husband was getting off at the next rest area. I couldn't read or even look at the scenery passing by. I just sat in the passenger's seat with my eyes closed and tried to distract myself by listening to music.

After the wedding, I ate the meal at the reception. I barely made it back to my hotel room in time to throw it all back up. Then I had the drive back home to look forward to.

—*Michelle Davis-Dash, MD*

∽

My second pregnancy with my daughter was absolutely the worst. Pretty soon after I found out I was pregnant, I developed significant morning sickness. It lasted for most of my pregnancy.

GI PRO TIP: Keep It Down

No one likes to vomit. It's perfectly awful. When you're pregnant, and uncomfortable already, vomiting can just about put you over the edge. Here are some food remedies that might help you to avoid vomiting.

- Experiment with diet changes. Keep a food diary to see what foods, and what times of the day are associated with the fewest symptoms.
- Consider toast, cereal, ginger biscuits, or crackers in the morning before getting out of bed. Then, rest for 20 minutes in bed before you start your day.
- Eat bland foods that are high in carbs and low in fat, such as mashed potatoes, bread, rice, and pasta.
- Try cheese or nuts before bed.
- Sip clear fruit juices, frozen juice pops, ginger ale, seltzer, other carbonated beverages, water, or ice chips during the day. You should drink at least 2 liters of fluids over a 24-hour period.
- Some warm beverages to try include:
  - Warm water with a squeeze of fresh lemon and a little honey
  - Warm water with peppermint, sugar, or honey
  - Warm water with 1 teaspoon of fennel seeds
  - Herbal tea with ginger or chamomile
- Chew some fennel seeds.
- Some women find that drinks that are too cold, tart, or sweet can worsen nausea and vomiting—avoid them!
- Eat small meals or snacks every two to three hours instead of three regular large meals.

- Eat foods high in vitamin B_6, such as brown rice, avocados, bananas, fish, corn, and nuts. Alternatively, speak with your doctor about a B_6 supplement: 25 milligrams, 3 times per day.
- Avoid fried, greasy, or spicy foods.
- Consider separating eating and drinking by 20 to 30 minutes.
- Make sure you're eating enough fiber—through cereal, dried fruits, or supplements.

The following lifestyle changes might also help.

- Get enough rest, sleep, and relaxation.
- Consider purchasing acupressure or sea-sickness wristbands.
- Join a pregnancy sickness support forum.
- Speak to a sympathetic listener.
- Don't blame yourself for your symptoms.
- Take care of yourself.
- Consider time off from work.
- Speak with your doctor.
- Carry a "sick kit" when you go out, packed with tissues, "sick bags," water, mints, or hard candies.
- Keep your bladder empty.
- Don't swallow excessive saliva. Spit it out, and do frequent mouth washing.
- Wear clothes that keep you feeling comfortable.
- Avoid crowded or overly warm places.
- Go out for a walk.
- Keep rooms well ventilated.

—Stacey Ann Weiland, MD

The timing of the "morning sickness" was really off, though. My nausea was the worst in the evenings. During most of that pregnancy, I pretty much consistently threw up my dinner.

The hardest part about that was that I couldn't keep down a good meal, and I couldn't keep down my prenatal vitamins.

On top of all of that, I had a very hectic work schedule. I really tried my hardest to stay hydrated at all times. On most days, my goal was survival—never mind feeling great and thriving!

Because of the severe morning sickness and vomiting, I couldn't consume enough iron. In the beginning of my pregnancy, my hemoglobin level was 16 gms/dl. By week 36, it had dropped to close to 8 gms/dl.

This was very scary because if my hemoglobin level dropped to 8, I wouldn't have been allowed to deliver at the birth center with the midwifery team I had selected. To make matters worse, I knew that if I bled a lot during my delivery, I might have needed a transfusion.

Fortunately, I supplemented my diet carefully at the end of the pregnancy. The biggest additions I made were a lot of spinach and eggs and trying to cook things in a cast iron skillet. My midwife also prescribed a slow release iron pill that was more easily tolerated in terms of the GI symptoms I had been having. My hemoglobin levels stayed just high enough, and my delivery went smoothly. It worked out well.

—Sigrid Payne DaVeiga, MD, a mom of 11-year-old and 6-month-old sons and a 6-year-old daughter and a pediatric allergist with the Children's Hospital of Philadelphia, in Philadelphia, PA

Get a Pregnancy Massage

Massage is a great way to treat yourself, reduce stress, ease muscle tension, and feel calm, relaxed, and pampered. Designed specifically for pregnant women, prenatal massage uses cushions that take pressure off the lower back and pelvic area. A massage gives you a chance to lie down, relax, and take your mind off of your morning sickness.

Some chain massage therapy centers offer pregnancy massage. But before you make an appointment, make sure the therapist has completed a prenatal massage training program. The American Pregnancy Massage Association is a good place to look for a therapist. Learn more here: **AMERICANPREGNANCYMASSAGE.ORG.**

If you don't have the money—or energy—to pay for a massage, for goodness sakes, ask your partner for one! A gentle neck and back rub or foot rub will help to melt away your tension, and it may help you to connect with your partner. Plus, it will likely make him feel great to be able to do something to make you feel better.

When I was pregnant with my older son, I started throwing up around week 10. I literally puked until I delivered that child. I had HG. At first, I thought it was just very bad morning sickness. But by week 13, I knew it wasn't normal.

I threw up pretty much every couple of hours while I was awake. One of the most challenging things about it was that it was so random. I would need to throw up suddenly, without warning. It could happen at home, in my car on the way to work, or at the hospital. Or probably all three.

I tried everything that anyone suggested. My doctor prescribed Phenergan and Zofran. These prescription medications did nothing for my nausea.

Mommy MD Guides-Recommended Product
Preggie Drops Plus with B_6

According to some studies, vitamin B_6 might help reduce nausea. Customers asked for Preggie Drops with vitamin B_6, and Three Lollies delivered.

Preggie Drops Plus with B_6 contain 10 milligrams of vitamin B_6. They're all-natural and drug-free. Three Lollies recommends not taking more than six lozenges or chews a day if they contain vitamin B_6.

A container of 21 pieces costs $5.50. Buy them at drugstores, retailers, or at **THREELOLLIES.COM.**

My pharmacist suggested trying metal acupressure bracelets. They didn't help.

Someone said I should try lemon. I put lemon juice in my water. It didn't work.

A friend recommended hypnosis. I tried it for six weeks. It didn't help my morning sickness, but I did learn how to hypnotize myself!

In the end, I just learned to cope with it.

I identified all of the spots along my commute where I could safely pull over to throw up. I also learned where all of the bathrooms were in the hospital and in all of my favorite stores.

My coworkers learned that it was better for them not to use the bathroom I usually threw up in—lest I throw up in the hallway if the bathroom was occupied. They put a sign that said "Dr. Brown's Restroom" on the door.

I stopped eating some foods that I found were really not too good the second time around: yogurt, other dairy foods, and pineapple. I remember thinking, "Never going to eat that again!"

Everywhere I went, I packed a toothbrush, toothpaste, and breath mints. At some point, you figure it out, and you move on. I survived. I was in my residency program, and I couldn't stop working. You do what you have to do. There's no stopping; you just have to keep moving forward.

Despite my severe morning sickness, I missed only two work days. The other days, I puked and kept on going.

—*Carrie Brown, MD*

I think most women with HG have some embarrassing vomiting stories. I know I do.

Once I was in the middle of patient rounds at the hospital. I knew I was about to vomit, and I couldn't hold it in. I said, "Excuse me, I'll be right back," and I dashed out of the room.

I made it to the bathroom and locked the door. As I vomited, the toilet seat fell down on my head. It startled me, and I screamed!

My residency-mates heard me and thought that something was terribly wrong. They ran around outside, banging on the bathroom door, frantically searching for the hospital key so they could rescue me. I kept trying to stop puking long enough to yell, "I'm okay!"

I'm still friends with many of them, and we laugh about that story to this day.

—*Carrie Brown, MD*

❧

At one point during my pregnancy, I vomited up blood. I went to the emergency department. Sometimes when you throw up so violently, you can tear blood vessels in your stomach or esophagus, and they bleed.

The emergency physician's advice? "Stop throwing up. It's bad for you."

Now why didn't I think of that?

—*Carrie Brown, MD*

DR. RALLIE'S TIP

When I first started taking my prenatal vitamins during my pregnancies, I began having morning sickness. I'm sure I would have had the morning sickness even without the prenatal vitamins, but the two became forever linked in my mind. To this day, just thinking about taking one of those giant pills makes me feel queasy and gaggy.

I think most pregnant women have had the experience of eating or drinking a particular food or beverage that made them vomit, and for the rest of their lives, those foods and beverages will have the power to stir up a little nausea. It's like a morning sickness flashback. For me, it's spiced tea and peanut butter. Although my youngest son is now a teenager, the faintest whiff of spiced tea or peanut butter will send my stomach into major spasms!

Chapter 5

Headache

Headaches are very common in pregnancy. In fact about 20 percent of moms-to-be develop a migraine during pregnancy.

Why? For several reasons. First, you're probably avoiding caffeine, and caffeine withdrawal can cause a headache.

Also, hormonal changes cause increased blood volume, even around your brain. This can trigger headaches. You might be feeling more stress, especially because you're coping with morning sickness. Certainly, stress can cause headaches. Any number of things may be wrecking your sleep. And lack of sleep might be making your head ache.

A challenge of pregnancy headache is you can't take very strong medicines to find relief. Hopefully, some of these remedies will stop the pounding.

JUSTIFICATION FOR A CELEBRATION

The feeling after a headache has passed—when you suddenly realize your head is no longer throbbing—is a truly wonderful sensation.

I had migraines from about week 16 to 22. I bought an ice gel cap, which is sometimes called a "headache hat," from Amazon. It worked wonders.

Because bright lights triggered my migraines, I avoided light and always wore sunglasses during the migraine.

I took acetaminophen (Tylenol) during pregnancy. Sometimes I took 50 milligrams of Benadryl. I'm not sure if it was the drug or the sedation that helped. Sleeping the migraines off always seems to help me—if I can get to sleep!

A few times when I had horrible migraines, I took Fiorcet, which is a combination of butalbital, acetaminophen, and caffeine. (Talk with your doctor or midwife before taking any medications.)

—Rachel S. Rohde, MD, a mom of a six-year-old daughter and a newborn, an associate professor of orthopaedic surgery at the Oakland University William Beaumont School of Medicine, and an orthopaedic upper extremity surgeon with Michigan Orthopaedic Institute, P.C., in Southfield, MI

Do not undervalue the headache. While it is at its sharpest, it seems a bad investment; but when relief begins, the unexpired remainder is worth $4 a minute.

—Mark Twain

Even when I'm not pregnant, I get migraines. They started when I was 14 years old. Every day, I take a preventive medicine, and I take an abortive medicine to help stop a migraine once it has started.

Some women get fewer headaches during pregnancy. When I was pregnant, I was lucky. I didn't get that many headaches. Some headaches are caused by hormone fluctuations. When you're pregnant, your hormones go up and they stay up. They're not bouncing around as much as when you're having regular menstrual cycles.

For the few headaches I got, I simply took Motrin and Tylenol. Then I went to bed and slept it off. It's hard to cope with a headache—especially when you're pregnant.

—Rebecca Jeanmonod, MD, a mom of 12- and 8-year-old daughters and 11- and 8-year-old sons and a professor of emergency medicine and the associate residency program director for the emergency medicine residency at St. Luke's University Health Network, in Bethlehem, PA

During my pregnancy, I had moderate headaches, and I wanted to avoid pain medicine. I purchased an apple-scented candle because the smell of apples is believed to help with headaches, I would lay down in a dark room and light the candle. It did help to manage the pain—but it didn't completely resolve it.

—Jennifer A. Gardner, MD, a mom of seven-year-old son, a pediatrician, and the founder of an online child wellness and weight management company, HealthyKidsCompany.com, in Washington, DC

When to Call Your Doctor or Midwife

Having headaches during pregnancy is no fun, but fortunately, most are harmless. In some cases, a headache can be a sign of a more serious problem. If you have a migraine for the first time during pregnancy, or if you have a headache that feels unlike any you've experienced before, call your doctor to ask if you need medical attention.

Signs of a migraine include severe head pain, nausea, and sensitivity to light and smell.

Go to an emergency department immediately if your headache:

- Is sudden and explosive or includes a violent pain that awakens you from sleep
- Is accompanied by fever and a stiff neck
- Becomes increasingly worse, and you have vision changes, slurred speech, drowsiness, numbness, or a change in alertness
- Occurs after falling or hitting your head
- Is accompanied by nasal congestion, pain and pressure underneath your eyes, or dental pain

In your second or third trimester, headaches can be a sign of preeclampsia, which is a pregnancy complication caused by high blood pressure. Seek medical attention immediately if your headache:

- Doesn't go away or recurs often
- Is sudden and very severe

- Is accompanied by blurry vision, spots in front of your eyes, sudden weight gain, pain in your upper right abdomen, and swelling in your hands or face
- Is accompanied by nausea and vomiting

The following types of headaches warrant an immediate call to your doctor or midwife.

- New onset headache in a woman who doesn't usually get headaches
- New type of headache in a woman with a history of headaches

The following types of severe headaches and symptoms warrant immediate medical attention at an emergency department; do not delay getting treatment.

- Sudden severe headache unresponsive to over-the-counter medications
- Thunderclap onset of headache
- Weakness or numbness on one side of the body
- Visual changes, blurred vision
- Seizures
- Inability to talk, find works, or slurred speech
- Headache changing with posture
- Difficulty walking
- Altered consciousness
- Accompanying fever, stiff neck, or rash
- Headache following a head injury
- Inability to move one eye in certain directions

DR. RALLIE'S TIP

I had a sinus infection the entire third trimester of each of my three pregnancies, and they gave me terrible headaches. Working in a hospital, I was exposed to just about every germ imaginable. As your pregnancy progresses, your immune system actually becomes somewhat suppressed. This is good for your baby, ensuring that your body doesn't accidentally try to reject her as a foreign invader, but it does make you more susceptible to colds,

GI PRO TIP: Ease the Squeeze

Pregnancy can often be good news for migraine sufferers because many women report a gradual reduction in the number and severity of migraine headaches as their pregnancies progress. This phenomenon is directly related to gradually increasing estrogen levels.

Studies show that 11 percent of women report improvement in migraine headaches in the first trimester, 53 percent report improvement in the second trimester, and 79 percent report improvement in the third trimester.

Because their migraines are less severe, many pregnant women are able to stop using prescription medications and can treat their symptoms in ways that are safer for their babies. These include the following:

- Ice packs

*flu, and other illnesses. My sinus infections always seemed to
start with a cold, and after a few days of a runny nose and
sneezing, my sinuses would start to swell and hurt, and this led
to headaches. I took antibiotics for the sinus infections when my
doctor prescribed them. I drank plenty of water to help my sinuses
drain, and I could usually get a little relief by lying down for a
few minutes with a warm washcloth on my face. When all else
failed, I took Tylenol and a nap!*

- Warm compresses
- Massage (Even rubbing your temples, shoulders, and neck can help reduce the pain of migraine headaches.)
- Relaxation, such as deep breathing and meditation
- Biofeedback
- Recording in a diary and then avoiding the foods and activities that tend to trigger migraine headaches
- Avoidance of triggers, such as stress; foods like chocolate, aged cheese, peanuts, and preserved meats; and lack of sleep
- Regular exercise
- Regular meal times, to keep blood sugar levels stable
- Regular sleep patterns
- Good posture, especially during the third trimester when your belly is big

—Stacey Ann Weiland, MD

GI PRO TIP: ID Your Pain

Here are the characteristics of common headache types.

HEADACHE TYPE	HEADACHE LOCATION	ASSOCIATED SYMPTOMS
Migraine	Usually one sided and throbbing	Nausea, vomiting, and sensitivity to light, sound, and head movement, with or without aura, which are visual disturbances
Tension	Generalized pressure or tightness around the head	Unaffected by activity; episodic
Cluster	Usually on one side around one eye, but may radiate to other areas of the face and neck. Can be excruciating, with a penetrating pain lasting 5 to 180 minutes	Nasal congestion and a runny nose, eye tearing, eye reddening, facial sweating, and swelling, all on the affected side of the head
Analgesic Rebound Headache	Dull, constant headache, which is often worse in the morning	Occurs in patients who overuse analgesic (pain-relieving) medications

—Stacey Ann Weiland, MD

Dr. Jim's Tip
IS MORNING SICKNESS IN MY HEAD?

No! Even quite recently, morning sickness was largely believed to be psychological.

A study by Canadian researchers published in 2002 of 500 pregnant women compared their perceptions about morning sickness to their physical symptoms of nausea and vomiting. The scientists concluded that physical symptoms only explained 14 percent of how the moms-to-be felt. But other experts disagreed with the findings, saying the theory that morning sickness is in women's heads teaches women not to listen to their bodies.

While you should never let anyone tell you your symptoms are in your head, researchers have found that psychological treatments such as hypnosis can help (See "GI Pro Tip: Feel Very Sleepy" on page 33).

If you're not finding relief for nausea through the typical methods (sucking on Preggie Pops, eating smaller meals, sipping ginger tea, munching on soda crackers, avoiding exposure to food odors) you may want to turn to something like hypnosis.

A great wind is blowing, and that gives you either imagination or a headache.

—*Catherine the Great*

During my third pregnancy, I started getting migraine head-aches all of a sudden. It was awful. My doctor mentioned that niacin can cause headaches, and we realized it was the extra niacin in the prenatal vitamins that was doing it. The prenatals I was taking contained 200 percent of the recommended Daily Value for niacin.

I stopped taking the prenatals, and sure enough, my migraines went away.

—*Patricia S. Brown, MD, a mom of two daughters and a son and a psychiatrist at Columbia-New York Child and Adolescent Telepsychiatry and in private practice in Cresskill, NJ*

∽

I had a headache every day during my seond trimester. I found that taking Tylenol and Sudafed each morning helped. I didn't have a history of migraines, so I didn't think they were migraines, just pregnancy-related headaches. (Talk with your doctor or midwife before taking this or any medication.)

I also found that when I was busy, I felt better. Sitting home feeling sorry for myself wasn't the way to go! Working kept my mind off of my headaches.

—*Ann LaBarge, MD, a mom of four children and an ob-gyn in private practice at the Midwest Center for Women's Healthcare in Park Ridge, IL*

MommyTime | Eat High-Potassium Foods Like Bananas to De-Stress

An apple a day might keep the doctor away, but did you know that a banana a day might blunt effects of stress?

High stress depletes potassium, so eating enough potassium will refill your stores.

Bananas are a popular high-potassium food. Other good sources of potassium include sweet potatoes, prune juice, soybeans, spinach, rainbow trout, and cantaloupe.

Processed food is often low in potassium, so you're almost always better off preparing your own meals, if you're feeling up to it. Need ideas for preparing quick and easy, nutritious meals and snacks during pregnancy? You'll find lots of great recipes in *The Mommy MD Guide to Losing Weight and Feeling Great*.

Chapter 6

Heartburn

Once one actually feels the pain that is heartburn, you really understand why it got that name. Literally, it is a burning near your heart.

Heartburn is very common in pregnancy. About half of pregnant women cope with it. Ironically, many pregnant women find just when the nausea lets up, the heartburn kicks in. Some very unlucky moms-to-be have both nausea and heartburn at the same time.

Pregnancy heartburn can be caused by several things. First, the hormone progesterone slows digestion. Second, your growing uterus is crowding other organs in your abdomen, pressing on your esophagus. Third, your esophagus actually slackens during pregnancy.

We hope some of these tips will help you spell R-E-L-I-E-F.

JUSTIFICATION FOR A CELEBRATION

When "feeling the burn" makes you think about exercise again, rather than heartburn, it'll be a good day.

During my first pregnancy, I was plagued with terrible heartburn. Eliminating all fat during the last trimester was a big help.

—*Amy Baxter, MD, a mom of 18- and 16-year-old sons and a 14-year-old daughter; the CEO of* buzzy4shots. com; *and the director of emergency research, Scottish Rite, of Children's Healthcare of Atlanta*

During my pregnancies, I had terrible heartburn. The worst culprit was orange juice. I had to stop drinking it entirely.

I got vitamin C from my prenatal vitamins and from eating other fruit.

—*Eva Mayer, MD, a mom of a 12-year-old daughter and an 11-year-old son, an associate professor of pediatrics at Temple University, and a pediatrician with St. Luke's Pediatrics Associates, in Bethlehem, PA*

During my first pregnancy, coffee gave me heartburn. I stopped drinking coffee then, and I still very rarely drink it, although it's been a long time since I was pregnant. It was one of those things like Pop-Tarts that pregnancy turned me off of. If I'm someplace where tea isn't available, I'll have a cup of coffee, but that happens fewer than five times a year.

—*Rebecca Jeanmonod, MD, a mom of 12- and 8-year-old daughters and 11- and 8-year-old sons and a professor of emergency medicine and the associate residency program director for the emergency medicine residency at St. Luke's University Health Network, in Bethlehem, PA*

DR. JIM'S TIP
IS MORNING SICKNESS MAKING ME DEPRESSED?

Maybe! Morning sickness can certainly affect your quality of life. In one study, researchers screened 230 pregnant women for anxiety and depression and also asked about their nausea and vomiting symptoms. They found that high scores of morning sickness had a significant correlation to anxiety and mild depression.

In another study of 367 pregnant women, researchers found that women who experienced severe nausea and vomiting had lower quality of life scores. Not surprisingly, feeling nauseous and having to head to the bathroom several times a day can have a huge impact on your appetite, stress level, your family life, and your ability to function.

If you think your morning sickness is leading to anxiety and depression, the first step to take is to get help for your nausea and vomiting symptoms. If you're not finding relief from morning sickness at home, see your doctor about possible drug remedies. While you're there, mention the stress, anxiety, or depression you're feeling. Your doctor may recommend talking with a therapist, or in more severe cases taking an antidepressant.

During my pregnancy, I had early waves of nausea and heartburn. My advice may be blasphemy today! I would cook full balanced meals and then tell my husband to pick me up fries and a Coke on the way home from work. Salt, grease, and soda settled my tummy. At least it was only for a few weeks.

—Katja Rowell, MD, a mom of a 10-year-old daughter, a family practice physician, and the author of Helping Your Child with Extreme Picky Eating and Love Me, Feed Me *at TheFeedingDoctor.com in St. Paul, MN*

⌒

Even when I'm not pregnant, I have heartburn. I've had it so bad in this pregnancy that it causes me to vomit foam. It also makes my stomach bubble and gurgle, and I get a terrible gnawing feeling.

Now that I'm pregnant, I have to watch what I eat very carefully. I find that fried foods make the heartburn worse. I can usually get away with eating simple starches, like rice, bread, and

When to Call Your Doctor or Midwife

Heartburn is so common during pregnancy that it's often thought of as a normal part of being pregnant. Normal, maybe. Comfortable, not.

When heartburn doesn't resolve on its own, you may want to talk to your doctor or midwife. She will likely suggest dietary and lifestyle changes, but when those don't do the trick, over-the-counter medicines are an option. But talk with your doctor or midwife before taking them.

Tell your doctor or midwife if your heartburn is severe, you spit up blood, or you have dark-colored bowel movements. These can be signs of blood in your digestive tract.

potatoes, and lean protein foods, including baked chicken and grilled steak.

—*Michelle Davis-Dash, MD, a mom of a five-year-old son, who's expecting another baby, and a pediatrician in Baltimore, MD*

⌒⌒

Many years after struggling with heartburn in pregnancy, I found that foods such as gluten, grains, and dairy can be triggers. I remember when the Atkins diet first came out, which severely restricts carbs such as grains. People who tried the Atkins diet found that their heartburn often went away. Now we know why.

A lot of people have food sensitivities. As physicians, the worst thing we can do is put these individuals on acid-blocking medications to mask their food sensitivities. That's just treating the symptoms rather than discovering the root cause.

—*Susan Wilder, MD, a mom of a 22-year-old daughter and twin 17-year-old girls, a primary care physician, and the founder and CEO of LifeScape Premier LLC, in Scottsdale, AZ*

⌒⌒

During my first pregnancy, my heartburn was worse than the nausea. I tried Tums, Zantac, and other antacids. But they didn't do much. I really got relief from ThroatCoat tea, which has slippery elm in it. It coated my esophagus and made the heartburn enormously better.

—*Amy Baxter, MD*

I had reflux during both of my pregnancies. It started around 20 weeks, and it lasted until delivery.

I tried to limit eating and drinking before bedtime, but that didn't always help. The over-the-counter medicines didn't work well so I ended up taking a prescription proton pump

GI PRO TIP: Cool the Burn

Most women want to avoid taking unnecessary medications during pregnancy. This is especially important between days 31 and 71 from your last menstrual period, because that's when your baby's organs are forming.

Heartburn can make you reach for some pharmaceutical relief like almost no other condition. Before you resort to taking medications, though, here are some things you can try:

Elevate the head of your bed. Your upper body—not just your head—needs to be elevated for heartburn relief. Do this by placing 6- to 8-inch blocks under the base of the bed or by lying on a 6- to 8-inch wedge-shaped foam rubber pad. The wedge should be long enough to extend from the head of your bed to your waist so that your entire chest is elevated.

Eat frequent small meals. Do this rather than eating three large meals each day.

Chew gum. Chewing sugar-free gum for 30 minutes after a meal has been shown to reduce the amount of acid in your

inhibitor pantoprazole (Protonix) twice a day, which helped a lot. (Talk with your doctor or midwife before taking any medications.) Incidentally, both of my children were born with a lot of hair, so maybe babies with hair causing heartburn isn't just an old wives' tale.

esophagus, possibly through a combination of greater production of saliva and faster gastric emptying.

Don't eat right before bed. Make sure you finish your last snack of the day at least two to three hours before you hit the sack.

Lie on your left side at night. Several studies have shown that sleeping on the left side instead of the right is associated with a higher esophageal sphincter pressure, which means less reflux.

Don't bend over after eating. Bending forward causes your gastric contents to flow from your stomach toward your esophagus. Also, if you need to tie your shoes or pick something up from the floor, don't bend over at your waist. Bend at your knees instead.

Avoid tight clothing. Wearing tight clothing can increase your intra-abdominal pressure, especially later in your pregnancy. Increased pressure in the abdomen can lead to acid reflux.

—*Stacey Ann Weiland, MD*

—Rachel S. Rohde, MD, a mom of a six-year-old daughter and a newborn, an associate professor of orthopaedic surgery at the Oakland University William Beaumont School of Medicine, and an orthopaedic upper extremity surgeon with Michigan Orthopaedic Institute, P.C., in Southfield, MI

I had really horrible heartburn in all three of my pregnancies. It was awful. Each time, it started early in the first trimester.

Pregnancy can contribute to heartburn in several ways. One, the increased belly pressure pushes the stomach acid back into your esophagus. Two, the higher levels of hormones cause your esophageal sphincter to loosen. That's the valve between your stomach and esophagus. Normally, it's nice and tight, keeping the food and acid in the stomach where it belongs. When the sphincter loosens during pregnancy, the acid can splash up into your more sensitive esophagus, and this causes the pain of heartburn.

During my pregnancies, my heartburn was so bad at night I could hardly sleep. My husband told me I made horrible gagging sounds in my sleep.

The only way I could sleep was if I propped myself up on pillows. By the end of my last pregnancy, I needed to be surrounded by eight pillows to sleep. There was no room for my husband in bed with me and all of my pillows. I had to move into the guest room!

—Rebecca Jeanmonod, MD

Write Thank You Notes to Loved Ones

It feels wonderful to receive a thank you note, but surprisingly, it often feels even better to send one. Expressing thanks and experiencing gratitude is one of the simplest ways that you can help yourself feel better.

We're grateful to have found plenty of research that supports this. (See what we did there?) In one study, published in the medical journal *American Psychologist*, participants were asked to write and then personally deliver a letter of gratitude. The result? Their happiness scores skyrocketed!

You might find that pregnancy offers you ample opportunities to give thanks. People love to give gifts to pregnant women! Your family, friends, coworkers, neighbors, and even people you barely know may be showering you with all things baby for weeks. Speaking of showers, you are likely to have a baby shower––maybe more than one. Therefore, you will have plenty of thank you notes to write.

Why not combine your thank you notes with a dose of craftiness? The creativity mixed with the gratitude may increase your happiness even more. Pinterest.com, canva.com, and etsy.com are all great sites for inspiration for thank you cards to buy or do-it-yourself.

Your heartburn won't stick around forever; it's a temporary discomfort. But your words of gratitude will last a long time.

> **Don't worry. Here's the thing I've learned about pregnancy. Everything feels like a crisis, and everything turns out to be heartburn.**
>
> —*Cammie McGovern, author of* Say What You Will

I really struggled with heartburn when I was pregnant with my twins. I ended up taking medication.

By the end of my pregnancy, my heartburn was so bad that I had to sleep sitting up in a chair. Needless to say, I didn't sleep well.

I was tired all of the time. I remember thinking, *I'm carrying twins. I'm running the equivalent of a marathon here—with two tiny parasites sucking the life out of me. Of course I'm tired!*

—*Susan Wilder, MD*

Sometimes when I had heartburn at work during my first pregnancies, I took Mylanta.

I took Tums when I was pregnant with my twins. I knew that my body's calcium needs were high, and Tums is a quick and easy source of calcium. The Tums did double duty: I could increase my intake of calcium and ease my heartburn at the same time.

—*Rebecca Jeanmonod, MD*

During my pregnancy, my heartburn was awful. It felt like I didn't have a functional lower esophageal sphincter (LES), which keeps stomach contents and acids from refluxing up, and causing heartburn.

Initially, I approached my heartburn with as little treatment as possible. I am of the philosophy that "less is more" when it came to my management of patients and my pregnancy!

So in the beginning, I tried diet modification, such as avoiding acidic foods (like orange juice) and having smaller portioned meals. It didn't take long for me to realize that this approach didn't help!

The next step in my "less is more" algorithm was trying antacids. Calcium carbonate is the primary ingredient. Although my OB prescribed pepcid/famotidine an H2-blocker, which blocks the synthesis of acid in the stomach and is

Mommy MD Guides-Recommended Product
Tums

Yes, it might sound obvious, but during pregnancy, nothing feels simple, so we are going to say this anyway. If you are bothered by heartburn, try good 'ol Tums. In addition to easing heartburn it will give you extra calcium to boot.

You can buy Tums at drugstores, grocery stores, and mass merchandisers and online, for around $4 for 48.

considered safe in pregnancy, I wanted first to try the calcium based antacids. I reasoned that my baby would benefit from the supplemental calcium.

However, I remembered from medical school that consuming too many antacids could result in milk alkali syndrome—and a long list of other symptoms. Milk alkali syndrome is when blood pH is above normal, and the calcium can't be metabolized adequately and could cause kidney damage.

So every morning, I would ration the recommended maximum dose (the number of tablets depends of the milligrams per tablet), which is printed on the label. As the day progressed, I'd reach into my plastic baggy of antacids, nibble on them as needed, and not have to worry about losing count of how many I have already consumed earlier that day.

Some days, I found that I didn't take all of the tablets that I had allotted myself. Other days, I found that I needed more than the recommended maximum dosage. On those days, I have to admit, I took an extra tablet and then I relied on the integrity of the maternal-placental barrier to buffer my baby.

My baby is now a healthy, lovable, almost-five-year-old little boy.

—*Edna Ma, MD, a mom of a 4-year-old son and an 18-month-old daughter, an anesthesiologist, and the founder of BareEASE pre-waxing numbing kit, in Los Angeles, CA*

DR. RALLIE'S TIP

I never had heartburn in my life until I was pregnant. I tried to control it with dietary changes—avoiding spicy foods and caffeine—but that was difficult because I was starving and eating all of the time. Eating a huge amount of food made the heartburn worse, stretching my stomach and pushing the food and acids back up into my esophagus, which causes burning and pain.

I still ate a lot (apparently nothing can kill my appetite), but I made myself eat smaller meals, even breaking up one meal into three mini-meals. I certainly wasn't denying myself any calories!

I discovered that drinking soft drinks helped my nausea, but it made my heartburn worse. Anything with bubbles seemed to stir things up.

> **The only thing I never have unless I'm pregnant is heartburn.**
>
> **—Jessica Capshaw, actress and costar of ABC's Grey's Anatomy**

Chapter 7

Constipation

Constipation is so common in pregnancy that about half of all moms-to-be deal with it. It's much more common in pregnancy than diarrhea.

Why? The same hormone that might be causing you heartburn, progesterone, is causing food to move more slowly through your system. This can cause constipation as well.

Constipation is also caused by a space issue. Your growing uterus is putting pressure on all of your organs, including your intestines, and this pressure grows as your baby does.

The following simple diet and lifestyle changes might help to get things moving again.

JUSTIFICATION FOR A CELEBRATION

Probably the only time in your life going to the bathroom will feel like a reason to celebrate will be that first post-pregnancy poop.

I had more constipation with my first pregnancy than I did with my second. What really helped me was to drink a few mugs of hot water with lemon. Within a few hours, the hot water hydrates and can act as a stool softener. The lemon helps peristalsis. In other words, it helps the intestine "move things along."

—*Rachel S. Rohde, MD, a mom of a six-year-old daughter and a newborn, an associate professor of orthopaedic surgery at the Oakland University William Beaumont School of Medicine, and an orthopaedic upper extremity surgeon with Michigan Orthopaedic Institute, P.C., in Southfield, MI*

I was really lucky during all three of my pregnancies. The only GI problem that I encountered was some sudden constipation during my second pregnancy.

I was in the middle of my second trimester when my family and I traveled to visit some of my husband's relatives in Germany. I'm sure the combination of the long flight, the pregnancy, and the very low-fiber German diet contributed to my problem. Those people don't seem to need any fruit or vegetables to get things moving! They must have iron intestines!

My husband and father-in-law went to the local pharmacy for me. My husband told the pharmacist about my problem, and that his "frau ist schwanger" (wife is pregnant).

The pharmacist sent home some kind of powder to mix in water. It was probably an osmotic laxative, which relieves constipation by increasing the water in your bowels. It took a few days before I finally had success.

I tell everyone who plans to travel to Europe, and

When to Call Your Doctor or Midwife

As many as half of all women experience constipation at some point during pregnancy. While there are plenty of do-it-yourself treatments, such as eating more fiber, drinking more water, and getting plenty of exercise, you can also opt for over-the-counter or prescription medication.

Most pregnant women will have minor constipation, but for some women, constipation will be a major issue. If you experience severe constipation accompanied (which means you haven't had a bowel movement in days) by abdominal pain, or if you have constipation alternating with diarrhea, or if you pass mucus or blood in your stool, it's time to call your doctor.

Constipation that lingers for three weeks or more may also be a sign of a medical condition.

It's a good idea to stay one step ahead of constipation. Left untreated, constipation can lead to unpleasant complications such as hemorrhoids and rectal prolapse, which is a condition in which part of the intestine pushes out through the anus from too much straining.

especially to those countries where the diet is basically meat and potatoes: Don't forget your fruit and veggies!

—*Stacey Ann Weiland, MD, a mother of a 14-year-old daughter and 9- and 7-year-old sons and an internist/gastroenterologist, in Denver, CO*

Mommy MD Guides–Recommended Product
Natural Calm

We live in a hurry-scurry, 24/7 life. We're always trying to do too much, too perfectly, too fast. The results of that? Stomach upset and stress. Many American adults are deficient in magnesium, which is an essential mineral that can help offset the negative effects of stress. Magnesium is very soothing to the gastrointestinal tract and has wonderful laxative properties. It can help boost brainpower, especially in people with memory problems. It's useful in alleviating a number of respiratory symptoms, and it can ease a migraine pronto.

—Rallie McAllister, MD, MPH, a mom of three sons and a family physician, in Lexington, KY

The best-selling magnesium supplement for nine years, Natural Calm supports heart, bone health, better sleep, and natural energy production. The variety of delicious organic flavors are naturally sweetened, vegan, gluten-free, and non-GMO. You can buy Natural Calm online and in health food stores for $15 to $16. Visit **NATURALVITALITY.COM/NATURAL-CALM** for more information.

MomMy TIME

Go Shopping at a Baby Store or Online

When you don't feel well, you might not feel like doing anything, especially anything that requires you to leave the house. Feeling sick and being isolated can take a toll on your mood.

Sometimes you might appreciate a diversion from feeling less than 100 percent. What better way to take your mind off things than shopping?

One study found that 62 percent of shoppers took part in "retail therapy" to cheer themselves up.

Another benefit of shopping for your baby is that it allows you to check necessary items off your "to buy" list. That wonderful feeling of productivity—and the sense that you're in control of at least one aspect of your life—can be a major mood mender.

If you shop in-store, you'll be enjoying the company of other people. Other people who are also pregnant to boot! The social interaction can boost your mood as well.

Here are some baby-specific stores you'll definitely want to visit: Pottery Barn Kids, buybuyBaby, Babies R Us, and Carter's.

Even if your morning sickness prevents you from leaving the house, you can still go on an online shopping spree. Here are a few sites from which to choose: **CARTERS.COM, GIGGLE.COM, ZULILY.COM, LITTLEME.COM, AMAZON.COM, AND TARGET.COM.**

GI PRO TIP: Let It Go

Constipation is a real pain in the butt. But fortunately, there are simple things you can do to help it pass.

Increase your fiber intake. Aim for 25 to 30 grams each day. But don't start taking this high amount suddenly, or you may suffer from significant bloating and abdominal discomfort. Increase your fiber intake gradually over several days to weeks. Good sources of dietary fiber include:

- Fresh fruits and veggies: Leave the skins on and start each meal with a salad featuring a variety of raw vegetables or fruit.
- Dried fruits, such as prunes and apricots: Consider a breakfast of dried fruits, stewed in a cupful of hot water. Mash the soft fruit and eat it, along with the juice.
- Beans, peas, lentils, legumes, nuts, sunflower seeds, and pumpkin seeds
- Bran cereals, whole grain bread, and brown rice
- Sweet potatoes
- Wheat bran: Add a couple of tablespoons to your cereal in the morning.

Hydrate. Here's how.

- Try to drink eight 12-ounce glasses of non-caffeinated fluids daily.
- Drink hot water with lemon and a tablespoon of psyllium husk before bed.

- Sip at least one glass of fruit juice every day, especially prune juice.

Exercise. Try to exercise at least three times a week for 20 to 30 minutes.

Some pregnancy-friendly exercises include:
- Walking
- Swimming
- Yoga
- Pilates
- Tai chi
- Indoor stationary cycling

For a two-for-one bonus, drink a glass of a warm liquid right after exercise.

Other remedies:

- Down a tablespoon of coconut oil or olive oil before each meal.
- Try taking a tablespoon of molasses every day.
- Use your gastrocolic reflex! It's the wave of muscle contraction that starts in your esophagus and travels through your entire gastrointestinal tract. When you eat, your body automatically sends signals to your colon to make room for the incoming food. Sit on the toilet after all meals.

—Stacey Ann Welland, MD

> **If people would take care of their body and cleanse their colon and intestines, their problems would be pretty much eliminated.**
>
> —*Dr. George C. Crile*

Throughout my first pregnancy, I was really constipated. During my second pregnancy, my doctor recommended a brand of prenatal vitamins that also has a stool softener in it. I thought that it was helping, and I was sure of it one morning when I forgot to take my prenatal vitamin. I took a regular vitamin instead, and all day long I felt like I couldn't poop. That convinced me!

> —*Sonia Ng, MD, a mom of two sons and a pediatrician and expert in sedation at Children's Hospital of Philadelphia Pediatric Care at Princeton Health Care System in Princeton, NJ*

DR. RALLIE'S TIP

To ward off constipation, I try to eat the right foods. Fortunately, I enjoy eating cruciferous vegetables, such as kale, broccoli, cabbage, and collard greens. These nutritional powerhouses are all high in fiber, which helps to prevent constipation.

As a bonus, these veggies also contain cancer-fighting

compounds called isothiocyanates (ITCs), which help destroy cancer cells, and sulforaphanes, which appear to strengthen the body's defense against cancer.

Findings from another study suggest that kale—and also my favorites garlic and strawberries—appear to protect the body from injury caused by nitrites. Found in hot dogs and other processed foods, nitrites are food preservatives that have been linked to the development of certain cancers.

Chapter 8

Thinking About Getting Pregnant Again

Right now, as your body is working overtime to grow your baby, the last thing on your mind might be having another baby. Or maybe that is on your mind—in the sense of I am NEVER going through this again!

We present these stories and tips of Mommy MD Guides who have been where you are, to offer you comfort and support.

JUSTIFICATION FOR A CELEBRATION

No matter how much you might worry that another pregnancy will be another go on the morning sickness carousel, just about any time that stick turns blue is a reason to feel great.

> **Out of difficulties, grow miracles.**
> —*Jean DeLa Breyére*

I had practically no morning sickness with my first pregnancy. That's probably why I thought I would sail right through pregnancy again. Boy, was I wrong!

If I had known then what I know now, I'm not sure I would have knowingly gotten pregnant again!

We haven't told our son yet that he's going to be a big brother. But he's seen me throw up so much, he might suspect something is up.

—*Michelle Davis-Dash, MD, a mom of a five-year-old son, who's expecting another baby, and a pediatrician in Baltimore, MD*

<hr />

My first son was a fertility baby—conceived through fertility treatments. We weren't really thinking about having another baby, let alone worrying about it, when suddenly I got pregnant again! It was probably a good thing that I wasn't able to think it through: *What are we doing here? Do I really want to live through that again?*

Astonishingly, I didn't throw up a single time during that second pregnancy. Because my second experience was so very different, I remember thinking, *Maybe this one is a girl!* Nope.

—*Carrie Brown, MD, a mom of 12- and 10-year-old sons and a general pediatrician who treats medically complex children and specializes in palliative care at Arkansas Children's Hospital, in Little Rock*

> **I knew life began where I stood in the dark,
> looking out into the light.**
>
> —*Yusef Komunyakaa*

My two pregnancies were very different. I had a lot of morning sickness with my first, but very little with my second. I think that because you're so busy with the second pregnancy, you don't have time to be sick.

I think in your first pregnancy, you're completely wrapped up in being pregnant. You're so very aware of every feeling and symptom. It's exciting and novel, and it's also scary and all-consuming.

During my second pregnancy, I was working hard juggling a career and raising my disabled child. The second pregnancy just didn't take on the same importance as the first. I just kind of got through it.

I didn't have any morning sickness in my second pregnancy. I wasn't even as tired. I was grateful for that because I remember thinking, *I don't know how I would deal with being that tired again.*

—Eva Ritvo, MD, a mom of 25- and 21-year-old daughters, a psychiatrist, and the founder of bekindr.com, a movement to bring more kindness to the world, using neuroscience as the foundation, in Miami Beach, FL

The toughness and strength of women really come out in pregnancy. Pregnant women will calmly go to a bathroom, puke, come back out, and get on with their lives.

I think if you laid out the adverse effects of pregnancy like a drug warning label—This condition will cause nausea, vomiting, hemorrhoids, varicose veins, heartburn, headaches, stretch marks, and more—no sane person would ever get pregnant! We throw all of that out of the window, go into complete denial mode, and get pregnant. And some of us do it again.

—*Susan Wilder, MD, a mom of a 22-year-old daughter and twin 17-year-old girls, a primary care physician, and the founder and CEO of LifeScape Premier LLC, in Scottsdale, AZ*

MommyTIME

Sit on Your Porch—or Someone Else's—and Do Nothing!

Your amazing, strong body is creating another human being. Let that sink in! Every second of every minute of every day during your pregnancy, your body is working on overdrive to create a new life. So anytime you're doing anything else—cooking, cleaning, working, reading this book—you're actually multitasking!

Consider this complete permission to sit on your porch—or anywhere peaceful, quiet, and safe—and do absolutely nothing. And smile because you're *not* doing nothing. You're building a baby.

> You are full of unshaped dreams. You are laden with beginnings. There is hope in you.
>
> —*Lola Ridge*

DR. RALLIE'S TIP

I found out I was expecting my third baby when my second baby was just five months old. It occurred to me that I might possibly be pregnant when I began experiencing some early-morning queasiness that felt remarkably similar to morning sickness. But I immediately dismissed the idea. Everyone knows you can't get pregnant while you're breastfeeding, using contraception, and too sleep-deprived to even think about romance.

Two twin packs of pregnancy tests repeatedly confirmed that I was indeed pregnant. My husband and I were simultaneously overwhelmed and overjoyed.

My morning sickness was persistent and predictable, but I didn't really mind it. With your first pregnancy, there's just no way to imagine how much love and joy your baby will bring into your life. By the time your're expecting your second or third baby, you realize that you're about to receive one of the most precious, amazing gifts that life has to offer. Joyous anticipation goes a very long way when it come to surviving morning sickness!

Index

Note: <u>Underlined</u> references indicate boxed text.

M

Ma, Edna, 6–7, 21, 93–94

Magnesium, benefits of, 100

Male morning sickness, 42

Martin, Noni, xvi

Massage, 65

Mayer, Eva, 49, 84

McAllister, Rallie, xvi–xviii, 100, 125–26. *See also* Dr. Rallie's Tips

Mental attitude, about morning sickness, 16, 23–24

Migraines. *See also* Headaches
from niacin, 80
pregnancy improving, 76
prevalence of, 71
signs of, 74, 78
treatments for, 72, 73, 76–77, 100
when to call your doctor or midwife about, 74–75

Milk alkali syndrome, 94

Mommy MD Guides. *See also specific Mommy MDs*
diverse stories of, xvii–xviii

Mommy MD Guides–Recommended Products
Natural Calm, 100
Preggie Drops Plus with B₆, 66
Preggie Pop Drops, 35
Preggie Pops, 17
Sea-Band Antinausea Bands, 41
Tums, 93

Mommy MD Guide to Losing Weight and Feeling Great, The, 81

MomMy Time
breathing technique, 25
buying yourself flowers, 32
eating high-potassium foods, 81
pregnancy massage, 65
pregnancy-safe yoga, 46–47
shopping, 101
sitting and doing nothing, 110
watching YouTube funny videos, 21
writing thank you notes, 91

Morning sickness. *See also* Nausea; Vomiting
causes of, 1
dealing with dismissal of, 7
dehydration from, 2, 54
depression from, 85
duration of, 1, 4, 5–6, 12, 16, 17, 22
effect on baby, 1–2
factors worsening, 2
gagging with, 3, 11, 22, 23, 39
as hereditary, 53
incidence of, 1
male, 42
mental attitude and, 16, 23–24
onset of, xv, 1, 4, 5, 8, 12, 22, 23
as pregnancy sign, 3, 22, 111
prenatal vitamins and, 4, 14, 69, 80, 84
protective evolutionary theory for, 6–7
as psychological, 79
remedies for
distraction, 6, 16, 21, 30
foods, 3, 4–5, 8, 9, 11–12, 15, 21, 30, 35, 54, 60, 79
fresh scents, 32, 44–45, 45

Prenatal vitamins
  headaches from, 80
  morning sickness and, 4, 14, 69,
    80, 84
  stool softener in, 104
  vitamin C in, 84
  vomiting from, 23, 53, 64
Prenatal yoga, 46
Protonix, for heartburn, 89
Proton pump inhibitor, for
    heartburn, 88–89
PsiBands, for easing morning
    sickness, 9
Ptyalism, xvii
  duration of, 27
  possible causes of, 27–28
  with severe morning sickness, 29
  symptoms of, 27, 29, 30, 32
  treatments for, 31, 33, 35
  when to call your doctor or
    midwife about, 29

R

Rectal prolapse, 99
Reflux. *See* Heartburn
Retail therapy, 101
Ridlan, for preventing vomiting,
    59
Ritvo, Eva, 4, 8, 9, 13, 16, 19–20,
    44–45, 53, 109
Rohde, Rachel S., 8, 39, 52–53,
    72, 88–90, 98
Rowell, Katja, 85–86

S

Salivation, excessive, 11. *See also*
    Ptyalism

Saltines, for easing morning
    sickness, 4
Sea-Band Antinausea Bands, 9,
    41
Shopping for your baby, 101
Sinus infection, 76–77
Sitting and doing nothing, 110
Sleep, for migraine relief, 72
Sleep position, for heartburn
    relief, 89, 90
Sleep problems, 11
  headaches from, 71
  from heartburn, 90, 92
Small meals
  for easing morning sickness, 8,
    31, 62
  for heartburn relief, 88, 93, 95
Smell sensitivity, xvii, 11, 40–41
  duration of, 37–38
  reasons for, 37
  remedies for, 39, 44–45, 48,
    49
  to specific foods, 37, 39, 40, 43,
    46–47, 49
  when to call your doctor or
    midwife about, 39
Social support, importance of,
    18–20
Strachan, Dina, 30
Stress
  breathing technique reducing,
    25
  headaches from, 71
  magnesium for, 100
  potassium-rich foods and, 81
  social support easing, 18, 20
Sudafed, for headaches, 80

with ptyalism, 29, <u>31</u>
with sinus infections, 77
for vomiting prevention, <u>62</u>
Weight gain, when carrying
    twins, 57
Weight loss
    from hyperemesis gravidarum,
        51, <u>58</u>, <u>59</u>
    from morning sickness, 2, <u>10</u>,
        <u>29</u>, <u>54</u>, 56, 57
Weiland, Stacey Ann, 98–100
    GI Pro Tips of (*see* GI Pro Tips)

Wilder, Susan, 3, 9, 40, 52, 87,
    92, 110

Y

Yoga, prenatal, <u>46</u>
YouTube funny baby videos, <u>21</u>

Z

Zofran, for nausea, 13, 52, 66

The Natural Way to Ease Morning Sickness!

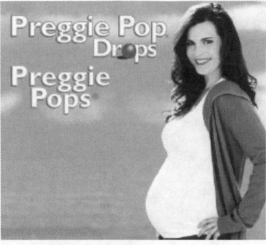

Preggie Pops

These naturally flavored lollipops and lozenges are specifically formulated for pregnant women. They work via a combination of essential oils, aromatherapy, and our unique delivery system. Preggie Pops also help alleviate dry mouth and provide comfort and energy during labor.

www.threelollies.com

866.773.4443

ALSO BY
MOMOSA PUBLISHING LLC

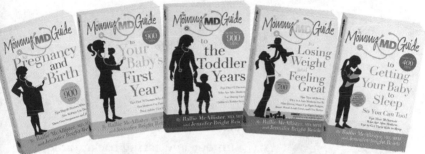

- Order our books online at many sites, including Walmart.com, Amazon.com, and MommyMDGuides.com

- Purchase them at bookstores nationwide

- Download them for your Kindle, Nook, or iPhone/iPad

• • •

Enjoy more Mommy MD Guides' tips on

The Mommy MD Guide to Pregnancy and Birth app.

Visit us at MommyMDGuides.com
and DaddyMDGuides.com.

COMING SOON!

*The Mommy MD Guides are hard at work on more titles in the series.
Keep a lookout for:*

The Mommy MD Guide to Keeping Your Baby Safe

About the Authors

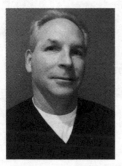

JIM PATHMAN, PHD, Dr. Pathman has a unique and caring background, which adds to his abilities in managing the Three Lollies. Long before the conception of Preggie Pops, Dr. Pathman identified his love of helping others feel better. As a very young adult, he helped treat autistic and emotionally challenged children. His dedication and devotion to the care of others carried him through both Masters and Doctoral degrees in the field of Psychology. To his credit, Dr. Pathman has always aimed at "helping people feel better." As a Psychologist for a large utilities company, Dr. Pathman helped both individuals and large groups identify and resolve conflict issues—helping to improve the workplace environment. As the director of a Behavioral Science program in a Family Practice setting, Dr. Pathman helps young healthcare providers become familiar with the psychological needs of their patients, and this means patients receive a higher level of care.

Currently, Dr. Pathman's energy is focused on the research, development, and production of Preggie Pops, Queasy Pops, and Three Lollies' growing line of products. His enthusiasm and devotion are unbeatable.

Finally, Dr. Pathman's most prized and coveted role is that of father and husband. He devotes countless hours and abundant energy and support to his 19-year-old daughter. As stated by his wife of 26-plus years, "Jim's dedication and devotion to all that he loves is the definition of his being." His daughter, on the other hand, describes him as "a Lollie of a Pop."

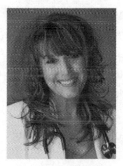

RALLIE MCALLISTER, MD, MPH

Dr. McAllister is a family physician and nationally known health expert. She is also a cofounder of Momosa Publishing LLC, publisher of MommyMDGuides.com and DaddyMD-Guides.com and the Mommy MD Guides book series. She is a coauthor of *The Mommy MD Guide to Pregnancy and Birth*, *The Mommy MD Guide to Your Baby's First Year*, *The Mommy MD Guide to the Toddler Years*, *The Mommy MD Guide to Losing Weight and Feeling Great*, and *The Mommy MD Guide to Getting Your Baby to Sleep*.

Dr. McAllister's nationally syndicated newspaper column, Your Health, appeared in more than 30 newspapers in the United States and Canada and was read by more than a million people each week.

A nationally recognized physician, Dr. McAllister has been the featured medical expert on more than 100 radio and television shows, including *Good Morning America Health, ABC News,* and *Fox News.* She's the former host of *Rallie on Health,* a weekly regional health magazine on WJHL News Channel 11 with more than one million viewers in a five-state area, and a weekly radio talk show.

A dynamic public speaker, Dr. McAllister educates and entertains audiences from coast to coast with her upbeat, down-to-earth delivery of the latest health news.

Dr. McAllister is the author of several other books, including *Healthy Lunchbox: The Working Mom's Guide to Keeping You and Your Kids Trim,* and the founder of PonyUP! Kentucky, a company that creates unique, equestrian-style handbags and accessories to raise money to support rescued and retired horses.

She is also a mother of three sons and a grandmother of three.